APHASIA IN CHILDREN

Under the Advisory Editorship of J. Jeffrey Auer

APHASIA IN CHILDREN

JON EISENSON, Ph. D.

Scottish Rite Institute for Childhood Aphasia
Stanford University School of Medicine

HARPER & ROW, Publishers

NEW YORK   EVANSTON   SAN FRANCISCO   LONDON

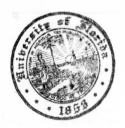

CONTENTS

Preface

This book, which perhaps might just as appropriately be called *Linguistically Retarded Children,* incorporates observations and research with children who were evaluated and treated at the Institute for Childhood Aphasia (ICA), School of Medicine, Stanford University. The ICA was established with an initial and continuing grant from the California Scottish Rite Foundation. We have also been fortunate in receiving support for our research studies in the form of a program research grant from The National Institute of Neurological Diseases and Stroke.

Aphasic children, though infrequent in number, represent a special population of perceptually impaired children who are seriously delayed in their onset and acquisition of language. However, there are so many other children with perceptual disturbances and lesser language delay, who resemble aphasic children in their psychological profiles and language development, that a book on their problems seemed to be needed. The author hopes that this book answers the need.

The approaches in the book, both for diagnosis and treatment, make use of materials in the literature that became available in the 1960s. The orientation basically is that provided by recent contributions of linguists and psycholinguists, as well as by speech pathologists and speech scientists who are interested in language acquisition. We hope that the therapeutic programs included in the book will serve to stimulate efforts along the same lines at other agencies that are concerned with children who are delayed in language acquisition and development. The author is grateful to the children who have been seen for diagnosis and treatment in the Institute for Childhood Aphasia and to the members of the Institute whose efforts contributed to the research and therapeutic approaches we have tried and refined.

Jon Eisenson

Normal Language Acquisition

With the knowledge of what constitutes the nature and range of normal language acquisition in the child, the student should be able to relate this information to congenitally aphasic and other children who are atypical in their language competence. We shall in this chapter highlight some features of language acquisition and indicate the stages at which differences between normal and severely linguistically retarded children begin to appear.

The capacity to acquire some form of speech, that is, to learn a linguistic code that normally employs distance-reception (hearing and vision), is a human species–specific function denied to very few human beings. These few include only the most severely mentally

Chapter 1

retarded, the severely perceptually impaired, and a very small number of nonrelating children (the nonverbal autistic). Almost all other human beings can acquire some form of language behavior, although the extent and complexity of this behavior varies considerably from individual to individual. The achievement is not denied to the blind, though they are somewhat later in language acquisition than the seeing; it is not denied to the deaf if we accept, as we should, the premise that visual signs can and do constitute a language code; it is not denied to congenitally aphasic children, though its onset is late and its development is retarded and in some respects deviant from normal children:

Most children learn to speak by ear; that is, they acquire speech through aural–oral means and learn an aural–oral system. Operationally, a child may be said to be speaking when he demonstrates through his production[1] that his utterances conform to the conventions of other speakers in his environment These conventions include the acquisition of a phonemic (sound) system, a morphemic (sound combining) system, and a syntactical, or grammatic, system (the combination of words into *strings,* or formulations, that approximate the utterances of older members of his environment). However, the child neither duplicates nor replicates. He approximates others, but ultimately learns to speak as a self in a way that identifies him as a self.

Criteria for Language Acquisition

Sometime between nine and eighteen months of age most children who will acquire speech utter their first true words. The first words are likely to be the designation-identification of persons or things, spoken only when the persons or things are actually present. Shortly thereafter, however, most normal children will begin to announce by naming what they wish to have present. So, "Mama," or "Dada," or "wawa" may be said by a child to have mother come, or an out-of-reach and perhaps out-of-sight doll or other play object, be handed to him. He has discovered the magic of speech. Before these pronouncements the child is likely to have learned a considerable number of words, or sentences with key

---

[1]We will assume, for the sake of ease of exposition, that we will be talking about a normal child with normal hearing.

words, and he may point to his nose, or place his hand on top of his head on command, or even play peek-a-boo with an admiring adult. Comprehension, with or without overt reaction, both precedes and exceeds production of language throughout life. To return for the moment to the child and his beginnings as a verbal member of his environment, we may describe this period as being one in which the following criteria are met:

1. The child understands and derives meaning from a conventionalized system of audible and/or visible signs (symbols).

2. The child without specific and direct training, understands verbal formulations to which he has not been specifically exposed. Thus, a child trained to "Where is the dolly?" but not to "where is the ball?" nevertheless understands and behaves appropriately to the second utterance. The child is listening *creatively;* he understands new word formulations based on what he has previously learned.

3. The child produces new verbal formulations (new strings of utterances), which are understood by listeners. He is now speaking creatively, his creations the products of the inventory of words and words phrases under his command.

The second and third criteria indicate that the child is capable of generalizing from specific words and utterances he has learned (been taught) directly to comprehension and production (generation) of an indefinite number of new formulations. In a very real and important sense, the child has become a self-generator of language. Somehow he has learned the rules used by those about him for verbal expression. He generalizes and frequently overgeneralizes linguistic rules, and applies them to what he hears and what he wishes to say.[2] Often the errors the child makes suggest that he is more rigid in his application of rules than are older speakers. Thus, *childs* may be used as a plural for *child,* and *sheeps* as a plural for *sheep.* Later on the child may learn that adults are people who have many exceptions in the way they speak and may become an "exceptional" speaker himself.

[2]See Chomsky, N., "The Formal Nature of Language," in Lenneberg, E. H. (1967, Appendix A), for a detailed exposition of the concept of generative language.

DEVELOPMENTAL LANGUAGE STAGES

Prelingual Stages

Although we began our exposition with the child's first words, we will now consider the prelingual stages in the development toward language. Before a child utters words with intent either to name or to bring about an event, he normally goes through a series of overlapping stages of vocalic and articulatory production. These early stages are universal; the kind of oral activity that the child engages in is not related to the language he will ultimately speak until, in fact, he is almost ready to speak and begins to "echo" some of the utterances to which he is specifically exposed in his environment. Although it has not been clearly established, we assume that the prelingual speech stages are necessary precursors for true speech. Carroll (1961, p. 337) suggests:

> Vocalizations, crying, cooing, and miscellaneous non-descript sounds of the first three or four months are probably most significant in that, in addition to exercising the maturing speech apparatus they make it possible for the infant to learn, through appropriate reinforcement, the instrumental, communicative character of vocal sounds, as when crying brings relief from hunger or pain.

Undifferentiated Crying

Babies normally announce their entry into the postuterine world with a cry. Those who fail to do so spontaneously (reflexively) are usually helped to crying by the services of the attending physician in the form of a sharp slap on the tender backside. The cry, if proper and lusty, provides some assurance that all is well. It is likely that the birth cry is a reflexive expression of the pain or discomfort the baby experiences by having to breathe entirely through his own efforts. For the first few weeks of his life, the baby is likely to cry in discomfort states and to sleep away much of the rest of his time. The cryings are undifferentiated; the nature or characteristics of the cries are not discernibly different in regard to the specific cause of the discomfort. The crying is essentially the same, regardless of whether the child is hungry, thirsty, too warm, too cold, or requires a change of linen. The crying may be described as shrill, nasal wailing.

Assuming that we are dealing with a normal, full-term baby, we consider the cries in the first few weeks as reflexive manifestations of physiological, internal changes. From the point of view of the oral (speech) mechanism, crying indicates that the respiratory, laryngeal, and oral mechanisms are functioning normally. The child is able to approximate his vocal bands, and he can set them in motion as he inhales and exhales. Any identifiable sounds produced during crying are likely to be nasalized vowels.

Some infants may vocalize in periods we would regard as comfortable, e.g., after a bath, or after a feeding and "de-bubbling." Such noncrying vocalizations are infrequent in children younger than one month. Comfort vocalization increases in the normal child beginning with the second month.

Differentiated Vocalization

Beginning with the second month crying, as well as other vocalizations, become more expressive and increasingly differentiated in regard to quality and intensity as well as to varying external conditions. An observant mother may note that a child may stop crying, if only for a moment, merely by her presence. The mother may also derive some meaning from the child's crying and identify one cry as a call for feeding and another as a call for a change of linen. The infant's crying begins to have a signal function. This, however, does not suggest intention on the part of the infant. It does suggest that the mother is associating the kinds of crying with the kinds of discomfort situations.

As we indicated earlier, vocalizations may also signal comfort states, so that the mother, as well as other motivated and observant adults, may recognize the child's state of being, his moods, and his irritabilities by the way the infant sounds. Although the child's vocalizations become increasingly differentiated, they are still essentially reflexive. The adult's inferences do not imply any intention on the part of the infant. At three or four months of age, the child may well begin to imply what the adult infers from the vocalizations.

Recent research indicates that brain-damaged infants can be distinguished from normal infants on the basis of latency period (time after receiving a painful stimulus) and the duration of crying as a response to a painful stimulus. Fischelli and Karelitz (1962, 1963) employed a rubber band snapping to the sole of an infant's foot as a stimulus to induce crying. They found that normal infants, including nine who were under 35 days of age, cried more readily than did abnormal (brain-damaged) infants. They also found that abnormal infants required more stimulation than the normals in order to evoke the same amount of crying. Furthermore, the cry of the brain-damaged infants was not as well sustained as that of the normal ones.

Cooing and Other Comfort Sounds

During the second and third month cooing, gurgling, squealing, and sounds that approximate consonants as well as a variety of vowellike sounds become part of the infant's inventory of vocalizations. At about 12 weeks vowellike cooing may be sustained for 15 to 20 seconds (Lenneberg, 1967, p. 128). The infant is now becoming quite proficient in his sound making which, incidentally, is not restricted to the speech sounds of the speakers in his home environment. Discerning adults may identify front vowels, those of see and man, as well as "oh," "uh," and "ooh." Consonants that closely approximate m, b, g, and k may also be identified.

Responses to Sounds

By four months of age the child begins to make definite responses, by vocalizations, cessation of vocalization, or change in body posture, to other human sounds and sound makers. The child, on hearing a speaker, turns in his direction. If the speaker is not readily in view, the child's eyes scan the area in search for the sound maker. If the child himself is busy vocalizing, his initial reaction is to stop as he begins to search. If his search is successful and the speaker is located, the child may then repond by smiling or cooing. Vocal play may be maintained by continued interchange between the child and an adult. Infant vocalization may be encouraged and reinforced by the stimulating presence of a vocalizing adult. The evidence also indicates that children deprived of such stimulation, e.g., children brought up in orphanages, do less vocalizing than children who are brought up and attended to at their own homes (Brodbeck and Irwin, 1946; Goldfarb, 1954).

Deficient Sound-Makers and Nonresponding Children

There are some children, few and fascinating, who are notably almost silent in their early infancy. They also show little, if any, response (differential behavior) to the presence or stimulating attempts of adults. Except for token whimpering, they do little crying and do not engage in sound play. Later, those who fail to acquire speech, as well as those who speak but in a manner quite different from their peers, may be identified as *autistic children*. In their parsimonious vocalizations as well as in their failure to respond to other human beings, they reveal that they are non-relating children. Though most of them are neither deaf nor in any usual sense mentally retarded, they continue to be silent children, who are not impressed by human sounds. In retrospect, parents of such children recall them as being good, quiet ones. After age two or three the "goodness" begins to become a cause of concern because along with the lack of normal vocal play there is also a failure to identify with speakers and a failure to acquire normal speech.

Babbling

Between three and six months, most infants spend an appreciable amount of time in vocal play. In the course of their vocalizations they may produce identifiable sounds and even identifiable sound combinations such as "bah," "ga," and "ng." Some of the combinations may be duplicated, e.g., "ga-ga."

During the same period the child shows increased awareness of persons in his environment, even when they may not be talking to him. So a child may squeal in apparent delight at the sight of his mother, in accepting a toy, or when removed from his crib to be placed in his playpen. He also begins to show sensitivity to "No-No" sounds, especially when they come from persons with whom he has come to associate warmth and acceptance. Sudden, loud sounds, regardless of source, are upsetting and likely to produce crying.

Babbling is an important milestone-stage in prelingual speech development. During this stage innate drives toward vocalization and sound play may either be reinforced or discouraged. The child's potential as a sound maker is now subject to external factors. The influences of his specific environment—how much, how, and when people around him talk—become determining factors in the child's future as a speaker. By six months of age most children seem to be aware that vocal play is pleasurable, as an accomplishment in itself and as a device, a form of behavior, that gives pleasure to others. If such pleasure is apparent, then the child has dual sources of reinforcement for his vocal play. Thus Lewis (1959) notes that though the forces that bring the child to babbling are innate, babbling is enhanced and sustained by the nature of the specific environment. A favorable environment, one that will sustain babbling and encourage further prelingual development, is one that includes attentive, responsive, but not overwhelming, adults.

By the end of the fifth or sixth month a discerning listener should be able to note differences between vocalizations of deaf and hearing children. Most of the differences will be in the responses the children make to other vocalizers. Although the deaf child may engage in spontaneous, self-initiated vocal play, his repetoire of sounds is not as varied as that of the hearing child. Lenneberg (1964) observes:

> . . . the total amount of a deaf child's vocalization may not be different from that of a hearing child, but the hearing child at this age will constantly run through a large repetoire of sounds whereas deaf children will be making the same sounds sometimes for weeks on end and then, suddenly change to some other set of sounds and "specialize" in these for a while. There is no consistent preference among deaf children for specific sounds.

In spontaneous vocalization the voice of the deaf child is not different from that of the hearing child.

Lalling

Between six and eight months of age most children engage in a considerable amount of self-imitation in their vocal play (lalling). Repeated syllables such as "da-da," "ga-ga," and "ma-ma" may be heard. Often these are produced with accompanying inflectional (intonational) patterns that resemble those of older speakers in the child's environment. The nature of the intonation may suggest that the child wants something to be done for him *now,* or that he is either pleased or displeased with what is being done. The child's "utterances" are no longer as random as they were in the babbling stage. He makes fewer sounds, but seems to make them with some suggestion of intention. He is now monitoring his productions, is definitely listening to himself, and is apparently in control of his efforts. Some of his duplicated sound combinations such as "ma-ma" and "da-da" resemble words and in some instances may actually be uttered as identification-designations of persons or things about him. However, very few children at eight months have any actual intention or assignment of meaning by their utterances. They may, however, begin to understand a few words and recognize "baby" and some names of their playthings.

Echolalia

About eight or nine months of age most normal children enter the echolalia stage of their prelingual speech development. They do not, however, give up their lalling and may even on occasion revert to babbling. The significant advance in the echolalic stage is that the child now begins to be an imitator of the speech-sound productions he hears. The early imitative efforts may at first seem to be somewhat wide of the mark, so that "ba-ba" may be the response to either "ma-ma" or "daddy," or both. Gradually, however, the approximations begin to be replications of what is presented to him. Imitative efforts may also be observed for what the child sees as accompaniments of the sounds. Thus a child may wave and orally produce "bye-bye" without intended meaning. Vocal intonation may also be imitated so that the child, in all but change in postural set for doing what he seems to be saying, sounds as if he is speaking.

If the child is not yet truly speaking, as he well may in another two or three months, he certainly is increasing his comprehension of speech. The child shows increasing evidence of making differential and appropriate responses to some utterances addressed to him. He may, for example, reach or look for his ball on hearing the word "ball." He may reach for or hug his doll on direction or in answer to the question "Do you want your doll?" extend his hands for it. Echolalia may well continue into the next stage, when the child begins to name some of the things of importance to him in his environment.

Identification Language

By the end of the first year some children begin to say their first true words. By the end of the first three months of the second year many children say their first words, and by the middle of the second year the vast majority of children who are destined to be members of the speaking species will have said their first words. However, because echolalic utterances are likely to continue, many children appear to have a much larger linguistic inventory than they actually have. Operationally, we may now say that unless appropriate behavior accompanies an utterance, e.g., reaching for an object if an utterance resembling its name is produced, the child is not really speaking. On the positive side we may say that any utterance, however wide the approximation for the "real thing," is true speech if appropriate behavior consistently accompanies it. So "da-da" may refer to either parent or be a general designation for an adult, if it is the utterance produced on the appearance of one of the parents or of any acceptable adult.

First words are usually reduplicated syllables such as "dada," "mama," or "baba." As we have indicated, they are produced as identifications or designations, as announcements for the presence of an event. The child at this stage, and when in the mood, may be able to obey verbal commands such as pointing to his nose when told "Show me your nose" or when asked "Where is baby's nose?" He may bang with his cup, spoon, or with his hand on the order to "go bang-bang." In this respect we should note that the child is identifying verbal events by appropriate behavior. The child who bangs his cup not "on command" but as a self-initiated act to get a game started, or, better, to get some milk, or who says "cup" or something that approximates "milk" in order to get some, has entered into a significantly higher level of speech.

True Speech: Anticipatory Language

By 18 months of age most children are able to employ a few words, and some/ children many words, to bring about an event, to make something happen that might not otherwise occur. We refer to this as *anticipatory language* for two reasons. First, the child, presumably on the basis of rudimentary inner language, appears to expect that something will happen as a result of his utterance. If the event does happen, he will show his satisfaction. If it does not happen, the child may repeat his utterance or cry to show his disappointment. Second, the child reveals by a postural change and by motor set that he expects something to happen and has prepared himself for it. So if he says "mama," he looks for his mother to come into view. If he says "dolly" or "wawa," he acts as if he is ready for one or the other. If he says "up," he usually readies himself to be picked up. Words thus used have the power of magic. The child gets what he wants, and usually the adult is happy to do the child's bidding.

Between 18 and 24 months most children increase their productive vocabularies from one or two words to vocabularies of from three to fifty words. Their comprehension vocabularies are, of course, considerably larger. Some children may have "collapsed" words that sound like two-word phrases, e.g., "babyup." A small percentage of children in the 18 to 24-month age group may actually have several two-word phrase-sentences such as "baby-nose" and "dolly-nose." The normal under-two age child shows rapid growth in linguistic competence and is now ready for the acquisition of much more complex verbal behavior.

Functionally, the child's single-word utterances are sentences. The meaning of the individual utterance is determined by the word (lexical unit) and by the way it is intoned. Thus, "mama," depending on accompanying intonation, may mean "Where is Mama?" "Mama, I want you here," or even "That's enough of you, Mama!" If we accept intonation as a form akin to syntax, then the child's variously intoned single-word utterances, if the intonation pattern follows the conventions (practices) of normal older speakers, constitute complete sentences. This parallels what adults do with such oral products as "Yes," "No," and "Uh-uh."

Children who are severely mentally retarded may not advance beyond the single-word or word-phrase identification language stage. A small percentage of retarded children may acquire some anticipatory language, single words or two-word phrase-sentences, which they employ to bring about events. Growth of vocabulary is slow, both for the comprehension and for the production of language. Lenneberg (1964, p. 159) sums up the relationship between mental retardation and language acquisition as follows:

A complete and total absence of speech and language is seen only in the lowest grades of idiocy. With a mental age (ascertained by non-verbal tests) of thirty to thirty-six months, primative stages of language development, such as a small vocabulary, are usually demonstrable. With advances in mental age, higher stages of language development are attained and a mental age of five years leaves no effect upon the essential principles of speech production or language comprehension, even though the content of conversation will obviously be restricted.

We should like to emphasize that retarded children not only have smaller vocabularies than their normal age peers, but have fewer meanings for the words they know. Abstract concepts may be beyond their comprehension.

Syntactic Speech

By age two most children have vocabularies of fifty to a hundred words or more. Some children will have names for all the familiar objects in their environment. The most distinctive achievement, however, is not in vocabulary growth but in the ability to combine words into phrase-sentences. Although most of these utterances may lack the conventional markers of syntax—the use of functional words (prepositions and conjunctions) and plural and tense endings—they nevertheless constitute functional sentences. The literal form of the words may comprise two nouns, e.g., "baby-milk" to mean "I want milk" or "Give me some milk," or an adverb and a noun as in "More milk." Functionally, any words used by a two-year-old may serve to indicate a variety of meanings. What matters is that the child is now using different words and combining them to indicate different meanings. Frequently, one word may be used recurrently as part of a pivot utterance (Braine, 1963) so that the child may produce such phrase-sentences as "Here dolly" and "Here ball" as well as "Baby here" and "Cup here." We may also have such utterances as "More cup" and "More up" or the same words in reverse order. The significance of this achievement is that the child is developing awareness of sentence sense and word order. In time, usually within the next year, the word combinations will be modified by grammatical markers, the use of functional words to "tie" and relate the other words, and the conventions of word order according to the verbal practices (syntax) of older speakers.

By two years of age half or more of the child's utterances are sufficiently intelligible to be understood by listeners who are not in regular and frequent contact with him. This, presumably, encourages continued efforts at word formulations. Of special significance at this stage is the child's ability to combine words in new formulations that he has not been specifically exposed to in his environment. So from the inventory of words he knows, he creates sentences that may parallel some he has been directly taught. Thus, if he learned by imitation to say "Tommy up," he may improvise "Dolly up" and "Ball up" as well as "Mommy up" or, as we have indicated, the same words in reverse order. The child now reveals an ability to generalize and to generate and has, in effect, become a creative speaker (the third criterion for language acquisition).

Syntactic development is delayed in the mentally retarded. Based on a study of 61 mongoloid children and 23 with other types of mental retardation, Lenneberg (1967, pp. 154–157) observed that mental retardates with IQ's of about 70 are about 18 months behind children with mean IQ's of 100 in regard to syntactic (grammatical) proficiency; those with IQ's of 60 are about five years delayed compared to normal children in regard to syntactic development. Lillywhite and Bradley (1969, p. 165) note that "accurate syntax in verbal expression is slow to develop in retarded children."

Furth (1966, p. 15) observes that deaf children are, in general, incompetent or deficient in language competence as judged by their difficulty in the mastery of sequential ordering and syntactic modification of words. As a general observation Furth notes, "Many persons whom we do not consider capable of complex intelligent behavior learn the language of our society better than the majority of pupils in our schools for the deaf."

Communicative Intent

Between two and two and a half years of age children want not only an opportunity to talk but also some evidence that they have responding listeners. If a child of this age says something he expects should be understood, he demands evidence of understanding. If the evidence—an appropriate response—does not take place, he is likely to show frustration rather than repeat his utterance as he might have before age two. The child is now speaking with communicative intent. In a very important and literal sense, the child is emerging as a *self* who demands recognition. Fortunately, the verbal formulations of the two-year-plus child indicate that he is now speaking syntactically, grammatically or agrammatically, according to the verbal habits (syntax) of the older members of his environment. He is using three- and four-word sentences which include prepositions, articles, conjunctions, and other syntactical markers. His vocabulary growth rate is great, probably greater than at any other period in his life. His phonemic productions are also closer to those of adults, with a marked reduction in infantilisms. Water is more likely to be "water" rather than "wawa," and generally the child's phonemic proficiency is usually good enough so that almost everything he says is deservedly readily intelligible.

By age three the child speaks for himself and becomes an *I*. He uses the pronoun "I," whereas a few months before he had referred to himself as "me." More generally, the child is able to distinguish between "I" and "me," and "me" and "you." He can usually transform the "you" in a question such as "Do you want your ball?" to an "I" by answering "I want the ball," or possibly "I want it." There are some children who fail to make such pronoun substitutions. Among these are the autistic children who continue, if they are speaking, to refer to themselves by the pronoun used to address them. Thus, an autistic child may respond to the question "Do you want a cookie?" with "You want a cookie," or with a verbatim repetition of the original question. This failure in transformation of pronouns may be interpreted as an underlying lack of the autistic child in developing a concept of *self*. It may also be an expression, as we believe, of the autistic child's *drive for sameness,* which is characteristic of his overall behavior. By maintaining linguistic sameness the autistic child may be maintaining his self-concept and keeping his concept of his world, however defective, under control.

Three to Four: The Emergence of the Individuolect

By three years of age most children can understand thousands of words and have a productive vocabulary that may reach or exceed a thousand words. Almost all of their utterances are intelligible. Syntax approximates that of adult speakers, so that little more than some of the niceties of complex-sentence production remain as a next level of syntactic achievement. Phonemic proficiency, however, is not complete, and lisping and lalling (w substitutions for l and/or r) are common. By age four most children have improved considerably in this aspect of speech development. Some may, in fact, be speaking much as they will as adolescents and adults except that happily they still vocalize as children.

The four-year-old is a mature speaker with well-established language and is now showing evidence of developing his own rhetorical style. He may have favorite words and even favorite and individual ways of turning a phrase. The four-year-old speaks for himself and in a manner that expresses his self. Although he shares a linguistic system with other speakers in his environment, he is beginning to adapt the system to himself. He is now developing his *individuolect*.

The mentally retarded child at four or five years of age may also demonstrate style in language, but it is one characterized by articulatory delay, a paucity of vocabulary, limited syntax, and little or no creativity. Perhaps this is because moderate to severely mentally retarded children are weak in generalizing and even more inadequate in generating language. Their models for imitation are slavishly observed. They learn what they are taught, rather than what they are taught may represent. Lillywhite and Bradley observe (1969, p. 164) that "the retarded child who learns and repeats long commercials from TV programs, yet remains unable to use simple language effectively for communicating with others, baffles speech pathologists." The difficulty, we suggest, with the kind of mentally retarded child referred to by Lillywhite and Bradley is that he is at the mercy of his memory. He does not process what he hears and recalls, but reflects the content, as does the autistic child, without thinking. He knows the words but not the rules, and so he echo-imitates, but does not creatively generate linguistic formulations.

The speaking autistic child has a style which, as we have indicated, is all too often reflection without thinking. We have known four-year-old autistic children who could repeat verbatim, and in order, a series of radio or TV commercials. Syntax is likely to show an absence of pronominal transformation, so that the child uses the same pronoun when talking for himself as he does when he is addressed. The child may also echo-repeat statements made to him when engaged in an activity comparable to one in which the statement was first made. He may say "Very good, Johnny" when putting a block in place, if this is what was said earlier by someone else. Words may be used perseveratively, and neologisms may take the form of newly created words, or conventional words given unconventional designations. Thus a "mooer" may refer not only to a cow, but to any four-legged animal about the size of a cow, and a "meower" or a "meow" for any animal about the size of a cat.

Acquisition of Sounds: Phonemic Development

At about six months of age the infant, in his vocal play, produces some sounds and sound combinations that the adult identifies as belonging to his language system. At about eight months, the child begins to repeat syllables and word forms that closely resemble the adult's. The child's first words may sound like those spoken by adults or may be his own "inventions" of sounds that are easy to produce—"ma-ma" or "da-da." As the child learns to say more words, and even when he produces his word-phrases or two- or three-word sentences, it becomes apparent that lexical (word) and syntactic proficiency are more advanced than his articulatory (phonemic) proficiency. Between ages two and five, children show great variability in phonemic development. Some, especially girls, may be quite proficient by age three or four, and many have adult-level proficiency by age five. However, most girls do not level off in phonemic control until about age six or seven, and boys until about age seven or eight.

Children's errors in phonemic production and in phonemic control are not random or chance products. The child's first words are built of the sounds he can control—produced at will rather than as evocations in vocal play. These sounds are likely to include nasal consonants, labial (lip sounds), and vowels. The young child also engages in reduplication, possibly as an expression of normal perseverative behavior. Thus, with the sounds he is able to control, the child builds his inventory of first words. A word such as *mama*, which combines a nasal bilabial and a vowel, presents no problem. *Mama* is a "natural" in terms of phonemic proficiency as well as in opportunity for reinforcement. The word *dada* for daddy represents simplification through vowel reduplication. It is easier to say something twice than to say it once. *Dolly* may become "deedee" because of consonant and vowel duplication. The consonant /d/ is controlled before /l/. A *kitty* may be pronounced "kicky" because /k/ is usually controlled before /t/. The pronunciation of "bummy" for *bunny* may be explained by the substitution of the bilabial /m/ for the tongue-tip nasal /n/; it is easier to produce two bilabials in a word. In fact, the pronunciation "bubby" for *bunny* is not unusual.

As the child matures, usually first in auditory discrimination and then in articulatory control, he will begin to make distinctions between sounds that are phonemically similar. As we indicated, by age seven or eight the great majority of children reach what is essentially adult level of phonemic proficiency. In general, the process of phonemic development is one characterized by progressive differentiation. Almost all children can detect fine shades of differences before they can themselves produce them. A child may persist in his "kicky" for *kitty*, but reject this pronunciation from an adult; he may still produce "wawipop" at age five but resent such an offering from an older person. What the child is demonstrating by this apparently inconsistent language behavior is that at age four or five he has better phonemic discrimination, and so better expectations in regard to his listening, than he has motor control over his own productions. In a year or two, his motor control will be much improved, possibly because of a well-developed motor-kinesthetic auditory feedback loop. He may, according to the point of view of Liberman (1957, pp. 117–123) and Luria (1966, p. 102), begin to perceive speech according to the way he produces speech sounds. "Speech is perceived by the articulatory stimulus and the events we call perception . . ." (Liberman). The child then will perceive speech as he himself articulates the equivalents of what he hears. Whether or not this is indeed what takes place, an examination of the diagram of the brain (Figure 1, Chap. 3) will suggest that the proximity of the motor area for articulate speech to the temporal area for speech reception may well account for the establishment and interdependence of articulation and speech hearing.

Defective Articulation

Defective articulation is the most prevalent of speech disorders among children and is especially so among the mentally retarded. Lillywhite and Bradley observe (1969, p. 97) : "By far the most typical articulation pattern presented by the mentally retarded child is one of immaturity." As a general rule of thumb, we are likely to find that the mentally retarded child is proficient in articulation consistent with or somewhat below his mental age rather than with his chronological age. The most conspicuous type of error is that of sound omission. However, substitutions and distortions are also frequent. Errors of omission when they occur in final positions in words may represent syntactical deficiency—an absence of grammatical markers—rather than an inability to produce the sound per se. This would almost surely be the case if a sound is appropriately articulated in an initial position in an utterance, but omitted in a final position.

Some of the errors of articulation may be associated with the slower-than-normal development of the organs of articulation, or with poor motor control. Others may be the product of associated hearing loss, which has a much higher incidence among the mentally retarded than in nonretarded children.

Deafness is, of course, associated with difficulties in articulation. The profoundly deaf child is likely to be completely inarticulate unless he is trained by an oral method. Children with high-frequency deafness are likely to have serious difficulty with the production of sibilant and plosive consonants. Those with low-frequency deafness usually have difficulty with vowels, nasals, and semivowel sounds (l and r).

Cerebral-palsied children, as a total population, are seriously delayed in all aspects of language development. Many, even though they may not be mentally retarded, are markedly delayed and defective in articulatory proficiency. Irwin (1952) found that cerebral-palsied children at age five and a half are at the articulatory proficiency level of normal 30-month-old children. The problem of the development of articulation in the cerebral-palsied population is often complicated by hearing loss of both a peripheral and central nature.

Speech Readiness

An examination of the speech stages in Table 1 will reveal that the normal child appears to make great spurts in aspects of phonemic, morphemic, lexical, and syntactic acquisition at particular periods in his life. For example, we may note the large proportionate increase in vocabulary at about 30 months and the control of syntax at about 36 months. Consonant blends, which are not indicated on the table, are usually established between five and six years. These acquisition times may be considered periods of readiness in which basic skills of previous stages are incorporated, and the child is then "ready and able" for his next stage or level of development. Earlier we also indicated that regardless of the language the child will speak, most children acquire their first words at the beginning of their second year. Periods of readiness are opportune times for potential abilities (capacities) to become manifest abilities, provided that opportunity and conditions are right. For most children the essential right conditions are exposure to an older speaker and some reinforcement for their efforts. There is, of course, individual variation. For a given child the rate of progress after onset of speech will be determined by a combination of innate factors, such as the integrity of his neurological mechanism, his sensory capacities, and his native intelligence, and cultural factors that, at least until age three, are those which pertain within his own family. The factor of sex usually gives the girl some advantage over the boy until about age five. Bilingual exposure, especially for children from lower socioeconomic groups, is usually a negative factor. Position in the family usually gives a first child some advantage over younger siblings. However, the most significant environmental factors are appropriate stimulation and good models for identification with others, proficient speakers.

TABLE 1. Maturational Milestone, Motor Correlates, and Language Development

Age	Speech Stage	Motor Development
12–16 weeks	Coos and chuckles	Supports head in prone position; responds to human sounds by turning head in direction of sound source
20 weeks	Consonants modify vowel-like cooing; nasals and labial fricatives are frequently produced	Sits with support
6 months	Babbling, resembling one syllable utterances; identifiable combinations include "ma," "da," "di," "du"	Sits without props, using hands for support

Age	Speech Stage	Motor Development
8 months	Lalling and some echolalia	Stands by holding on to object; grasp with thumb apposition
10 months	Distinct echolalia which approximates sounds he hears; responds differentially to verbal sounds	Creeps efficiently; pulls to standing position; may take a side step while holding on to a fixed object
12 months	Reduplicated sounds in echolalia; possible first words for identification; responds appropriately to simple commands	Walks on hands and feet; may stand alone; may walk when held by one hand, or even take first steps alone
18 months	Has repertoire of words (between 3 and 50); some two-word phrases; vocalizations reveal intonational patterns; great increase in understanding of language	Walks with ease; runs; can build two-block tower; begins to show hand preference
24 months	Vocabulary of 50 or more words for naming and for bringing about events; two-word phrases of own formulation	Walks with ease; runs, can walk up or down stairs, planting both feet on each step
30 months	Vocabulary growth proportionately greater than at any other period in life; speaks with clear communicative intent; conventional sentences (syntax) of three, four, and five words; articulation still includes many infantilisms; good comprehension of speakers in his surroundings	Can jump; stand on one foot; good hand and fingers coordination; can build six-block tower
36 months	Vocabulary may exceed 1000 words; syntax much like that of older persons in his surroundings; most of his utterances are intelligible to older listeners	Runs proficiently; walks stairs with alternating feet; hand preference established

| 48 months | Except for articulation (phonemic production) the linguistic system is essentially that of the adults in his surroundings. He may begin to develop his own "rhetorical" style of favorite words and phrases | Can hop on one foot (usually right); can throw a ball to an intended receiver; can catch a ball in his arms; can walk on a line |

Source: Adapted from Lenneberg, E. H., *Biological Foundations of Language*, New York, Wiley, 1967, 128–130. By permission of John Wiley & Sons, Inc.

REFERENCES

Braine, M. D. S., "The Ontogeny of English Phrase Structure," *Language*, 39, 1963, 1–13.

Brodbeck, A. J., and Irwin, O. C., "The Speech Behavior of Infants without Families," *Child Development*, 17, 1946, 145–156.

Carroll, John B., "Language Development in Children," in *Psycholinguistics*, Saporta, S., ed., New York, Holt, Rinehart and Winston, 1961, 331–345.

Fischelli, V. R., and Karelitz, K., "The Cry Latencies of Normal Infants and Those with Brain Damage," *Journal of Pediatrics*, 62, 5, 1963, 724–734.

Furth, H. G., *Thinking Without Language*, New York, Free Press, 1966.

Goldfarb, W., "Effects of Psychological Deprivation in Infancy and Subsequent Stimulation," *American Journal of Psychiatry*, 12, 1954, 102–129.

Irwin, O. C., "Speech Development in the Young Child," *Journal of Speech and Hearing Disorders*, 17, 3, 1952, 269–279.

Karelitz, K., and Fischelli, V. R., "The Cry Thresholds of Normal Infants and Those with Brain Damage," *Journal of Pediatrics*, 61, 5, 1962, 679–685.

Lenneberg, E. H., "Language Disorders in Childhood," *Harvard Educational Review*, 34, 2, 1964, 152–177.

———, *Biological Foundations of Language*, New York, Wiley, 1967.

Lewis, M. M., *How Children Learn to Speak*, New York, Basic Books, 1959.

Liberman, A. M., "Some Results of Research on Speech Perception," *Journal of the Acoustical Society of America*, 29, 1957, 117–123.

Lillywhite, H. S., and Bradley, D. P., *Communication Problems in Mental Retardation*, New York, Harper & Row, 1969.

Luria, A. R., *The Higher Cortical Functions of Man*, New York, Basic Books, 1966.

Perception and Perceptual Functions Underlying Language Acquisition

We shall use the term perception as the process by which an individual organizes and interprets sensory data he has received on the basis of his past experience. In essence, perception implies an act of categorization according to which stimuli are taken in, identified, sorted, and given individual meaning. Perception for language, whether it is written or spoken, necessarily deals with a series or sequence of stimuli that have temporal order, that is, stimuli that are extended in time. In the discussion that follows we will be concerned with the perception of those auditory stimuli (events) that constitute speech. A primary and fundamental aspect of perception for speech is to differentiate and, however broadly, to categorize speech

Chapter 2

events from other environmental auditory events that simultaneously stimulate, or may stimulate, the respondent.

Perceptual Responses

The initial response to a perceptual experience is internal. It is, as Hebb (1966, p. 257) indicates, a mediating process which may or may not produce overt activity. We may perceive that a particular automobile is a sports car, a station wagon of a given type, or a taxi, without doing anything (make no differential motor response) in regard to the perception. We may hear a name called or hear a child or an animal "cry" and, according to circumstance, do something or do nothing. Unless we take the position that *doing nothing* is an appropriate motor response, we would conclude that perception is an intake process for which appropriate responses may be internal or external. When it is external, we then may use the term perceptual-motor process.

WORKING ASSUMPTIONS RELATIVE TO PERCEPTION

On the assumption that the individual has an intact sensory and motor system, which implies an intact neurological mechanism, then, depending upon the maturation and individual inventory of experience, there are several factors that affect and determine the perceptual process. We shall consider those about which there is common, if not unanimous, agreement among psychologists.

Selectivity

Perception is a selective process. We do not perceive everything that may come to us within a sensory field. Ordinarily, we respond to those events that have some priority or importance for us at a given moment. Thus, it is possible to hear the voice and the words of the person for whom we are listening rather than the person who is talking to us, or to see only one face in a crowd though our sensory system may have taken in many.

Factors that determine selection include *set* (we perceive what we are prepared or set to perceive), *drive, motivation, training,* and *cultural values.* The factors of drive and motivation need no explanation at this time, except to note that these may be negative, that is, there may be negative factors for us not to perceive. Training determines how we perceive cloud formation, automobile noises, or human noises. Bachelors, either because of motivation or training, may not be as adept at distinguishing a cat's crying in the darkness of the night from that of a baby's crying. Cultural values as well as training may determine the perceptions and both the covert and differential overt responses of parents to a baby's crying. Our knowledge (training) and our motivation determine whether we perceive or merely hear a foreign speaker when we are traveling abroad, or when at home where foreigners may be present.

Discrimination

With the possible exception of figure-background discrimination, the discrimination of objects, or of any pattern of events, is established through learning. Our capacity for making discriminatory responses increases with experience and learning.

Categorization

In our definition of perception we indicated that perception is a process of categorization. We may then ask, "Where did the first category that permits an individual to make additional categorizations come from?" We accept, as a basic assumption, that a normal organism is born with some innate categories and develops some categories with maturation. Thus, specifically in regard to speech, the infant is born with a capacity for making broad categorical responses between speech and other auditory (nonspeech environmental) events. As the infant matures his capacity for making finer discriminative responses permits him to establish sound (phonemic) categories for the language or languages to which he is exposed. Thus, our assumptions are that the normal infant has innate categories when he is born, as well as the capacity for developing additional categories according to his opportunities and experience.

Perceptual Defense

Some stimuli (events) may have unpleasant or painful associations for us, and may distress us or evoke anxiety when we are exposed to them. To avoid, at least unconsciously, such distress or anxiety, we tend to raise our threshold of awareness and so establish perceptual defense. Bruner (1957) suggests another related basis for the development of perceptual defense. Perceptual defense may occur

. . . first, through a failure to learn appropriate categories for sorting the environment and for following its sequences, and second, through a process of interference whereby more accessible categories with wide acceptance limits serve to mask or prevent the use of less accessible categories for the coding of stimulus inputs.

Bruner's notion has, we believe, important implication for the brain-damaged child. We conjecture that such a child may initially not have the capacity for making the discriminations between speech and nonspeech auditory events, and, when with maturation some basic categories are acquired, they may be so broad as to be essentially nonfunctional for speech perception. However, the broad, crude categories, once established, may continue to interfere with further perceptual categories. So, because of his perceptual defense, he may block out speech even though his cerebral system has matured enough to make him capable of auditory perception for speech.

Proximate and Distance Reception

Observations of the normal development of an infant reveals changes from proximate to distance reception, from an initial dependence on sensory intake of proximate (close to or in contact with the body) events to those which are at a distance from him. Our distance receptors—the eyes, ears, and nose—permit us to receive, perceive, and relate to the events of the world we cannot touch or taste. Some children, the autistic, seem to have difficulty for distance reception and so relate through direct body contact. Those who have visual or auditory impairments may need correction or assistance for distance reception. However, unless they also have central (brain) damage, they are able to integrate and perceive whatever they are able to receive.

The acquisition of speech is dependent on the capacity for distance reception. An impairment for distance reception, other than reduced sensory intake, and related impairment in the ability to integrate and make differential responses to distant stimuli will prevent the child from learning to speak. This, as we have suggested, may underlie the nonverbal, autistic child's failure to acquire speech.

Sequencing

In our opening statements about perception we indicated that perception for language necessarily requires that the individual must be able to deal with a series or sequences of events. The stimuli that constitute linguistic events, whether oral or written, occur in a sequence or order. The order, as we shall see later, is not altogether random but, within limits, is predictable. To be able to deal with linguistic events, and so to acquire normal language behavior, the infant and young child must be able to maintain the order of stimulus presentation in mind as the sequence is produced. The infant who succeeds in repeating a sound complex, even if it is as brief as "da" or "ma," demonstrates that he has learned to sequence two sounds, and to utter them as a single-syllabic combination. In learning to use a given linguistic system, in acquiring a spoken language, the young child somehow learns that some sequences or combinations of sounds are likely to occur while others just do not occur in a particular language. Perhaps when he is mature, and if he studies language systems, he will realize that some combinations do not occur in direct sequence because they are simply too difficult for the articulators to manage in a flow of utterance. If he is a bilingual child, he may also learn (become aware of) some things about sound (phonemic) sequences that he may have long practiced, that is, some sound sequences are practiced in one linguistic system but not in another, or in some parts of an utterance but not in all parts. He may learn that American and English speakers combine the sounds k + l, g + l, or p + l at the beginning of a word or at the end, though not precisely with the same effect, as in *club, cycle, glad, single, play,* and *apple.* However, d + l is not likely to occur at the beginning of a word, but often does at the end *(ladle, saddle)*. The sequences *dn* and *dv* will be reserved for foreign-looking words or names. By two years of age most children also learn, or at least begin to practice, word order according to the language or languages they speak. Thus a child who speaks any of the standard varieties of English may, before two years of age, have uttered either *pretty girl* or *girl pretty*, but it will not be long before he habitually says *pretty girl* if he speaks English, and reverses the order if he is saying the same thing in French. Bilingual English–French children will learn both word orders as they acquire two linguistic codes. We assume that as a child acquires a language, he somehow acquires the rules for the language. By applying these rules, for sound order and word order, his task in sequencing verbal content is facilitated. A rule, whether or not we are conscious or aware of its existence, permits us to anticipate or to guess as to what we may be responding to at a given moment in the light of a past response. It—a rule—also permits us to anticipate the next event. The important effect is that it no longer is necessary to load, or overload our minds with a greater number of events than we can easily process. We begin to "remember" even before the event has occurrd. Of course, what we begin to remember is the anticipated event. Then we count on feedback to confirm or reject the impression.

Sequencing is involved in memorization of content and in reproducing an order of events toward a particular objective. We memorize telephone numbers, addresses, social security numbers, and others that our culture and economy make it convenient for us to reproduce readily. We memorize how to operate appliances that require an order of pushing buttons and/or twisting dials. To imitate or initiate a given action that calls for more than a single movement requires an ability for sequencing. Each step we take, each time we bring hand to mouth or to some other organ, calls for sequencing. Probably the most complex of all sequencing acts is that of articulation in speech. For articulation we must assume that the unit for sequencing is an entire utterance. Normal persons, even allowing for normal hesitation phenomena or so-called disfluencies, speak in syllabic flows. We could not articulate in flows if utterance were controlled only by the preceding sound. We know that adults who suffer brain damage, with or without aphasic involvements, may have impairments in the control of a series or sequence of intended (nonreflex) movements. Such impairments are dyspraxias. When they disturb spoken utterance, they are oral dyspraxias or, if severe, oral apraxias. We believe that most expressive or productive disturbances in developmentally or congenitally aphasic children are really oral dyspraxias and, as such, an impairment in motor sequencing for speech.

PERCEPTUAL FUNCTIONS BASIC TO LANGUAGE ACQUISITION

Before we proceed to our discussion of perceptual disfunctions related to brain damage, and particularly to those brain-damaged children designated as aphasic, we will restate and list some basic intake (perceptual) functions for language acquisition. In order for a child to acquire (learn and produce) an oral language code, he must have the following capacities.

1. He must be able to receive stimuli that occur in a sequence or order.

2. He must be able to hold the sequence in mind, to hold the sequential impression, so that its components may be integrated in some pattern. This may be achieved either by memory or by the application of a rule plus memory.

3. He must be able to scan the pattern from within so that it may be compared with other stored patterns or other remembered impressions.

4. He must be able to respond differentially, to assign meaning on some level, to the identified pattern or impression.

5. In order to speak he must have an oral-articulatory system, or an equivalent manual system if he is deaf, to produce a flow or sequence of movements that constitute an utterance, audible and/or visible.

Sensory and Motor Involvements and Perception

As a general observation, we believe that limitations for the reception of sensory stimuli do not in themselves interfere with perception, provided the stimuli are received. Thus, peripheral hearing loss or visual refractory defects do not impair perception once the stimuli have been received so that they can be processed by the central nervous system. To be sure, unless the limitations are corrected by an adjustment to the loss—getting closer to the source of sound, having an aid to amplify sounds, making distance adjustments to the visual stimuli, or having properly fitted glasses —intake will be difficult, and there may be problems related to such difficulty.

We believe that the combination of peripheral *and* central impairment certainly aggravates the problem. This we sometimes find in developmentally aphasic children who present evidence of mild-to-moderate peripheral hearing loss. We also suspect that this may be an underlying problem for nonverbal infantile (primary) autistic children.

Perceptual Disfunctions

In determining possible perceptual disfunctions in children who cannot report verbally whether or how they have received or organized stimuli presented for input (intake), we must resort either to conjecture or to the interpretation of experimental investigations. The first approach, conjecture, assumes that we know as "fact" what we accept in theory. What we know as fact in regard to the brain damaged comes, for the most part, from acquired impairments in adults. As a result of fairly recent investigations we have gathered a considerable amount of information about breakdown in auditory perceptual functioning in adults. For the most part, the observed data are well reconciled with theory. We even know something about distorted perception in adult schizophrenics. By analogy we make assumptions for children. However, analogies may often be misleading. We need to be mindful of the differential effects of the time of onset of pathology on developmental processes. Thus, Eisenberg (1964, p. 68) observes that injury before speech acquisition "is even more devastating than similar injury in the adult." According to Eisenberg (1964, pp. 68–69), an early injury to the brain, pre- or postnatal, might impair

. . . an elementary psychological function, the lack of which could then distort subsequent development. Thus, complex functions, the anatomical equipment for which might otherwise be intact, could have failed to evolve. Whenever the injury is such as to impair the development of the capacity to symbolize (language) all subordinate functions which are ordered by language will develop less optimally and all patterns of social interaction will be grossly impaired.

If we resort to experimental investigations, we necessarily work on the assumption that the individual understands the task and the required response he is expected to make. We can, of course, train the child to make the responses, and so reduce the margin of error in our interpretation of what the child actually does.

However, we can by no means be certain that the child does indeed understand, and so the possibility for error must always be entertained. Earlier we indicated that dyspraxic involvements may make it difficult for a child, or for an adult for that matter, to express his intake in the form expected for a normal perceptual-motor activity. Thus, as Birch and Lefford (1964, p. 46) report, some brain-damaged (cerebral-palsied) children who make erroneous block-design reproductions are able, nevertheless, to choose a correct reproduction over their own product when directed to identify the one that most closely resembles the model. We have made a similar observation on aphasic children in regard to Bender-Gestalt figures.

Despite all of these precautions, we believe that there are some perceptual disfunctions which underlie the impairment for language acquisition in the developmentally aphasic child. For the present, let us consider the developmentally aphasic child as *brain different* and, therefore *perceptually different*. As a general and introductory observation we will state that as far as language acquisition is concerned, perceptual disfunctions may occur as a result of an impairment of any of the input processes considered in our summary statement above. Broadly stated, a perceptual disturbance for spoken language may be present because of the child's inability to organize sensory–auditory events even though "received," to hold the events in mind, and to scan them and compare them with others stored by the central nervous system. Perceptual disfunctions may also be a manifestation of categorical impairment. This may be on the basis of an absence or inadequate number of basic or innate categories from which further categories may be developed. Categorical development for phonemes (the sound system of a language) may also be impaired if the child does not modify his primary categories to permit the development of useful discriminations. If, for example, the primary category for sibilant sounds is so broad as to include all *s*, *sh*, *th*, and *f* sounds, he will be unable to make the necessary discriminations from what he hears to respond differentially to speech that includes these sounds. If this is indeed the case, he will derive little meaning out of what he hears. At the other extreme is the possibility that the child's categories are too narrow, too restricted, and too rigidly set. Thus, the child may have too many categories for functional sound discrimination. The *s* in words such as *see, sue, its,* and *pest* are somewhat different in duration and somewhat different in lip position, each determined by its context within the verbal utterance. Even more so are the *t*'s in *too, let Tom, get that,* and *letter.* However different allophonically, by the age of two almost all children "perceive" the /s/ sounds and the /t/ sounds as categories that encompass each of the varieties. If a child's categories are discrete, he necessarily has to overload his storage system with more individual sounds than he can readily recall and match as he is exposed to speech. If we bear in mind that no two persons articulate the same content in precisely the same manner, or that no person articulates precisely the same way twice even for the same content, we can appreciate the impairing implications of a precocious rigidity of sound categories. A child with such categorical involvement will be limited in his perceptual development for speech. He would, we conjecture, be considerably more impaired than a child who can read only if the print type and size are the same as the first printed words to which he was exposed.

Auditory Discrimination for Sequential Content

Spoken utterance, as we indicated earlier, consists of sequences of sounds. The order in which they occur is in part determined by the phonemic rules of the given linguistic system (see our earlier discussion on sequencing, pp. 26–27). However unwittingly applied, unless we followed rules that permitted us to anticipate and to make correct guesses as to what we are hearing, it is extremely unlikely that any human being could literally hear (listen) and separately identify each sound in a flow of utterance. Nevertheless, it is necessary to be a fast listener to keep up even with a slow talker.[1] How fast must a child be able to listen, to resolve what sounds he is hearing, and to keep the order of sounds in mind in

[1] In an article by Liberman et al. the authors point out that "speech can be followed, though with difficulty, at rates as high as 400 words per minute. If we assume an average of four to five phonemes for each English word, this rate yields about 30 phonemes per second. . . . Even 15 phonemes per second, which is not unusual in conversation, would seem more than the ear could cope with if phonemes were a string of discrete sounds" (p. 432). In essence, what these authors point out is that the ear can actually perceive more than it can possibly hear. This apparent inconsistency is related to the perceptual processing of speech sounds as part of a sound-decoding system which, as we indicated earlier, permits us to anticipate what we should be hearing, and in effect responding as if we did. For an expanded explanation, we recommend reading the provocative article by Liberman and his associates.

order to perceive the flow of sounds as speech? Unfortunately, we cannot answer this question directly. We can, however, present some evidence on aphasic adults as well as on aphasic children which indicates that auditory discrimination for sequential events is impaired and that there may be a generalized impairment for dealing with sequential events. We can also present some experimental evidence of how little time it takes for a normal perceiver to determine whether he is listening to two like events or two different events, and, if it is the latter, the order of presentation (reception and perception) of the events.

A rather common subjective response on first exposure to foreign-language speakers is that they seem to talk much more rapidly than we do. However, after increased opportunity for hearing the foreign speakers, even though we may not understand them, they seem to be speaking more slowly. This, of course, is not what takes place. It is much more likely that with added exposure, we begin to tune in and, in effect, become faster listeners. Recent experimental evidence supports our subjective impression about the effect of experience on our auditory perception. Broadbent and Ladefoged (1959) report an experiment in which they themselves were involved as subjects. They report that the time required for them to discriminate *piss-hiss* from *hiss-pipp* was reduced from 150 milliseconds (msec) to 30 msec after repeated trials of the task. Hirsh and Sherrick (1961) report that an experienced subject required an interval of 20 msec to report correctly (75 percent of the time) the presented order when two events, a light and a sound signal, are presented repeatedly in the same order. In a later experiment Hirsh and Fraisse (1965) report that naive subjects required about 60 msec for the same percentage of accuracy of performance when the discriminating decision had to be made on the basis of a single exposure of a light and a sound signal.

We have relatively few investigations on the ability of persons with verified brain damage in discriminating-sequencing tasks. The evidence, however, clearly indicates that cerebral pathology markedly impairs this ability. Efron (1963) compared a group of aphasic adults who had incurred left temporal lobe lesions with neurologically normal adults in their ability to make correct judgments as to the order of two 10-msec sound pulses that were markedly different in frequency. Efron found that the neurologically normal subjects required approximately 50 to 60 msec to make correct judgments as to the presented order of the sound pulses. In marked contrast, most of the aphasic patients required significantly more time, a few as much as a full second interval between sound pulses, before they could make correct judgments.

Lowe and Campbell (1965) performed an experiment with children much along the lines of Efron. The subjects ranged in age from 7 to 14 years, eight with aphasic (aphasoid) involvements and eight normals. The experimental serial-order task required that the subjects indicate the order of two 15-msec pulses, one at 2200 cycles per second (cps) and one at 400 cps. The time interval between pulses was varied in order for the investigator to determine the minimum time separation necessary for the subjects to indicate the correct order of the sound pulses. "Correctness" was assumed when the subjects reached a level of 75-percent accuracy. The range of interval time for the normal subjects was from 15 to 80 msec, with a mean of 36.1 msec. The range for the aphasoid children was from 55 to 700 msec, with a mean of 357 msec. The time interval difference between the groups was significant at the .005 level.

We need to be cautious about generalizing and applying the results of the studies we have just reported to aphasic children. On the face of it, signals such as discrete sound pulses and light flashes would seem to present a much simpler task for discrimination and sequencing (time-order determination) than would speech signals. However, signals of this sort do not permit of anticipation and "decoding" as spoken utterance might. The impairment for discrimination-sequencing, however, especially the appreciably longer time interval needed between signals for aphasic adults and children to make correct responses, is in keeping with clinical impressions. Aphasic children, as well as adults, seem to improve in comprehension of speech when the speaker reduces his rate of utterance. It is possible that this improvement is related to a reduction in quantity (bits of language to be processed) per unit of time. Investigations involving speech signals and spoken utterance are needed to give us the understanding we need about the perceptual functioning and impairments of the brain damaged for speech.

Discrimination of Speech Sounds:
Isolated Sounds vs. Sounds in Context

McReynolds (1966) utilized operant conditioning to investigate the ability of aphasic and nonaphasic children for speech sound discrimination. She selected three pairs of sounds, /m/ and zh/ʒ/, /s/ and sh/ʃ/, and /v/ and /z/ on the basis of distinctive feature theory (Jakobson, Fant, and Halle) according to which differences between phonemes can be expressed by the number of units or features of difference between two sounds. Subjects were trained to the task and were given up to 300 trials to make 10 consecutive correct discriminations. Only those subjects who succeeded were continued in the experiment proper. This required that the subject pull a lever to indicate which sound he was hearing. A correct choice was followed by a reinforcer—a bit of candy. An incorrect choice was left unrewarded. The experimental task was considered completed when the subject made a minimum of 16 correct responses out of 20 trials (80 percent correct), or completed 200 trials regardless of the number of correct responses.

In another phase of the McReynolds investigation, the subjects were limited to five presentations of the sound–lever association task for each sound and provided with a total of 100 trials to reach criterion on each task. The results indicated that the aphasic children made 70 percent correct discrimination for sounds in isolation compared with 75 percent for the normal children. However, one aphasic child failed to reach criterion in 300 trials and was excluded from the experiment. The aphasic group as a whole required 1640 trials compared with 1040 for the normal children.

When the key sounds were embedded in context, e.g., hamak [hamɑk] versus hashak [haʃak], or havak [havak] versus hazak [hazɑk], the aphasic children had increased difficulty in their initial efforts compared with the normal children. However, with repeated trials, discrimination and association improved. Ultimately, the aphasic children made 61 percent correct responses based on 2820ᵢ trials compared with 71 percent correct on 1860 trials for the normal children. McReynolds notes that "normal children not only perform more accurately within a fewer number of trials, but improve their performance more rapidly and more often than aphasic children." As a general observation, McReynolds notes

. . . the aphasic child requires more time (more trials) to respond reliably to a discrimination between speech sounds. Consequently, if he is given an insufficient amount of time he will in all likelihood respond erroneously, with the result that he would appear to be impaired in auditory discrimination ability.

There are several therapeutic implications in McReynolds' study. First, aphasic children do show an ability to learn to make discriminatory and associative responses. Second, they need more time and experience to demonstrate this ability. Third, in contextual speech, the aphasic children have increased difficulty but most, given enough opportunity, can make the necessary discriminations. However, we must appreciate that normal speech is not ordinarily limited to utterances of five phonemes.

Rosenthal (1970) investigated aphasic children and normal controls in experiments designed to study aspects of auditory temporal perception. Specifically, the experimental tasks required the subjects to make decisions on temporal order for speech and nonspeech signals. The subjects were eight aphasic and eight normal children, ranging in age from six to ten years. They were directed, after training, to indicate which member of a pair of auditory stimuli came first when the order of occurrences was randomly varied. Six different stimulus pairs were used: pure tone–noise; high tone–low tone; vowel "ah"–affricate "ch"; vowel "ah"–vowel "ee"; fricative "s"–fricative "sh"; and fricative "sh"–affricate "ch." These stimuli were selected in order to contrast certain characteristics of auditory signals—speech versus nonspeech and frequency versus temporal coding of information.

Rosenthal found significant differences in performance between normal and aphasic children as well as between different stimulus pairs. Under all stimulus conditions the normal children exhibited superior performance as measured by the minimum stimulus interval needed to resolve temporal order, that is, to make correct decisions as to which member of a stimulus pair came first. The normal children also had a higher percentage of correct responses at various interstimulus interval durations. In general, the pattern of response was similar for both groups, with errors increasing as the interstimulus interval decreased. The errors were not related with stimulus conditions based on a speech-nonspeech dimension. Interestingly, the easiest pair for the aphasic children was the vowel–affricate sequence; the most difficult pair was the fricative-affricate sequence. The respective mean minimum interstimulus interval was 64 msec for the vowel–affricate ("ah"–"ch") and 650 msec for the fricative–affricate ("s"–"sh").

When analogous speech and nonspeech pairs were compared (vowel–affricate versus pure tone–noise, and vowel "ah"–vowel "ee" versus high tone–low tone), the temporal order of the speech pair members was more accurately determined than nonspeech at shorter interstimulus intervals. Peak differences between these analogous pairs occurred at interstimulus intervals below 200 msec for the aphasic group and below 100 msec for the normal group. Comparisons of the fricative "s"–fricative "sh" and fricative "s"–affricate "ch" conditions indicated that the former pair, the members of which are distinguished on the basis of spectral energy, was more easily processed by aphasic children. This trend was reversed for normal children, who more easily processed the fricative "s"–affricate "ch" pair, in which the members are identical in spectral or frequency composition, but differ along a temporal dimension. This reversal was the only major difference in the pattern of responses between the groups.

The findings in Rosenthal's study indicate that aphasic children, even those who, though linguistically retarded are not nonverbal, require more time than normal children to resolve temporal order for auditory stimuli. However, Rosenthal notes:

It is significant that 7 of the 8 aphasic subjects were able to resolve the temporal order of at least one stimulus pair when the interstimulus interval was less than 100 milliseconds. This suggests that in those children tested, the auditory system is capable of processing most of the acoustic segments which comprise the speech signal. . . . It seems likely that the auditory temporal disorder which is presumed to underlie childhood or developmental aphasia serves to retard language development, but not to prevent its emergence completely. However, in older aphasic children, it is evident only under experimental conditions which test the limits of the auditory system.

Restated in nonlaboratory terms, we may observe that aphasic children are less efficient in auditory processing than normal children and continue to be somewhat slower and less efficient listeners than normal children, even after functional language is established. The therapeutic implications of this observation will be considered later in our discussion of training approaches for aphasic children.

Perception and Intersensory Stimulation

In our earlier discussion of proximate and distance reception we indicated that the perceptual development of the infant changes from initial dependence on proximate receptors to dependence on distance receptors. Birch and Lefford (1964, p. 48) observe along this line:

> In infants and young children, sensations deriving from the viscera and from stimuli applied to the skin surfaces appear to be predominant in directing behavior, whereas at these ages information presented visually or auditorily is relatively ineffective. As the child matures, the teloreceptive modalities assume an even more prominent position in the sensory hierarchy until, by school age, vision and audition appear to become the most important sensory modalities for directing behavior. Such hierarchial shifts are orderly and seem to be accompanied by increased intersensory liason in normal children.

Our emphasis for the present part of our discussion is on the development of intersensory reactions and perception in brain-damaged children. Birch and Lefford (1964, pp. 48–58) report the results of an intersensory study on a group of neurologically damaged (cerebral-palsied) children. The sensory systems studied were vision, kinesthesis, and haptic (touch and active exploratory movement of the hand). The stimulus items were blocks cut out as geometric forms. The subjects were directed to judge whether simultaneously presented stimuli in pairs were the same or different. The same blocks were used as the visual and haptic stimuli. The findings for the brain-damaged children were compared with those for normal children. Birch and Lefford note that for normal children, errors decrease with age for all conditions of intersensory interaction. For the brain-damaged subjects, despite considerable variability, the overall finding was that "at the very least, the emergence of such relationships appears to be delayed in the 'brain-damaged' children, a factor which may seriously limit possibilities for the normal utilization and integration of environmental information."

We cannot assume that developmentally aphasic children, who do not show the hard-sign evidence of the cerebral palsied, are equally impaired in their sensory-integrative functioning. The clinical evidence we do have suggests that some aphasic children tend to ignore auditory signals, but respond relatively well to visual signals. Almost all aphasic children perform much better on visual association tasks of the Illinois Test of Psycholinguistic Abilities (ITPA) (Kirk and McCarthy, 1968) than they do on auditory association. This, of course, is not an unexpected finding. If a child can perform up to or close to age expectation on the auditory tasks of the ITPA, he would not be aphasic. In clinical training that emphasizes visual perception in the early stages, aphasic children at the Stanford University Institute for Childhood Aphasia seem better able to accept and integrate visual-plus-auditory input than training approaches that begin with auditory discrimination. May (1967) utilized "nonsense" word discrimination, e.g., *hathak* versus *hatak,* and six-point random "nonsense" geometric forms, in an experimental investigation of auditory, visual, and combined discriminatory functioning. He found that auditory discrimination did not improve over 300 trials, but remained approximately at 65 percent correct discrimination. In contrast, visual discrimination improved from initial chance discrimination (50 percent) to 80 percent after 300 trials. This improvement was found to be significant at the 0.10 level of confidence. Combined auditory-plus-visual discrimination (simultaneous presentation of forms and nonsense words) was at 78 percent after the first hundred trials and remained at this level after 200 trials. After 300 trials the combined modality discrimination improved to 85 percent correct performance. The May study was an experimental investigation, which involved paired associates learning for two sets of artificial stimuli. It is different, therefore, from a "natural" situation in which a stimulus event may be recognized by its form as well as by its sound, e.g., a bell.

Wilson, Doehring, and Hirsh (1960) compared the performance of a group of 14 aphasic children who were classified as sensory aphasics with a group of nonaphasic children in an associative learning task. Specifically, the children were taught to associate four auditory stimuli that differed in quality and duration (a long tone, a short tone, a long noise, and short noise) with four visually presented letters of the alphabet. Eight of the aphasic children learned the task in about the same number of trials (fewer than 80) as the nonaphasic children. Six of the aphasic children failed to learn the task at the end of 80 trials.

The difference in learning ability within the aphasic group was unrelated to age, I.Q., or amount of hearing loss. [The investigator also notes that] informal observation on further training of the children who had failed to learn the task indicated that they were able to make the required discriminations among auditory stimuli, and that their poor performance was the result of a specific difficulty in learning to associate four visual stimuli with four auditory stimuli.

Berry (1969, p. 124) presents a possible explanation for some of the experimental findings and for the clinical observation that some neurologically handicapped children show impaired rather than enhanced perceptual functioning with multimodality stimulation.

We know that neural assemblies in several receptor systems may use the same routes; a child with CNS injury or deficit may be able to accommodate only impulses from one modality in a unit of time. In the normal child, on the other hand, the same neurones can participate in countless specific patterns of activity.

To summarize this phase of our discussion, aphasic children do not seem to show the severe degree of impairment for intersensory perception as do frankly cerebrally palsied children. Neither do they seem to do as well as normal children for integrating and perceiving multisensory events, and particularly for associating auditory and visual events. They seem to be more dependent and more proficient with visual input than with auditory input. Based on our clinical observation, aphasic children also seem to be able to accept auditory input when it is associated with the visual as the initially trained modality more readily than when training begins with the auditory.

REFERENCES

Berry, M. F., *Language Disorders of Children*, New York, Appleton-Century-Crofts, 1969.

Birch, H. G., and Lefford, A., "Two Strategies for Studying Perception in Brain Damaged Children," in *Brain Damage in Children*, Birch, H. G., ed., Baltimore, Williams and Wilkins, 1964, 46–60.

Broadbent, D. E., and Ladefoged, P., "Auditory Perception in Temporal Order," *Journal of the Acoustical Society of America*, 31, 1959, 1539.

Bruner, J. S., "On Perceptual Readiness," *Psychological Review*, 64, 2, 1957, 123–152.

Efron, R., "Temporal Perception, Aphasia, and Déjà Vu," *Brain*, 86, 1963, 403–424.

Eisenberg, L., "Behavioral Manifestations of Cerebral Damage in Childhood," in *Brain Damage in Children*, Birch, H. G., ed., Baltimore, Williams and Wilkins, 1964, 61–76.

Hebb, D. O., *A Textbook of Psychology*, 2nd ed., Philadelphia, Saunders, 1966.

Hirsh, I. J., and Fraisse, P. (1965), cited in "Central Institute for the Deaf Periodic Progress Reports," 8, 20, July 1964–June 1965.

———, and Sherrick, E. E., "Perceived Order in Different Sense Modalities," *Journal of Experimental Psychology*, 62, 1961, 423–432.

Kirk, S., and McCarthy, J., *The Illinois Test of Psycholinguistic Abilities*, Urbana, University of Illinois Press, 1968.

Liberman, A. M., Cooper, F. S., Shankweiler, D. P., and Studdert-Kennedy, M., "Perception of the Speech Code," *Psychological Review*, 74, 6, 1967, 431–461.

Lowe, A. D., and Campbell, R. A., "Temporal Discrimination in Aphasoid and Normal Children," *Journal of Speech and Hearing Research*, 8, 1965, 313–314.

May, M. Z., "An Experimental Investigation of Multimodal Discrimination Learning by Aphasic Children Utilizing an Automated Apparatus," Ph.D. dissertation, Stanford University, 1967.

McReynolds, L. V., "Operant Conditioning for Investigating Speech Sound Discrimination in Aphasic Children," *Journal of Speech and Hearing Research*, 9, 1966, 519–528.

Rosenthal, W. S., "Perception of Temporal Order in Aphasic and Normal Children as a Function of Certain Stimulus Parameters," Ph.D. dissertation, Stanford University, 1970.

Wilson, L. F., Doehring, D. G., and Hirsh, I. J., "Auditory Discrimination Learning by Aphasic and Nonaphasic Children," *Journal of Speech and Hearing Research*, 3, 2, 1960, 130–137.

Brain Mechanisms and Language Functioning

Our objective in this chapter is to present some basic information on the structures of the brain mechanisms that are related to language (speech) functions. We will consider such matters as localization of functions that underlie speech, cerebral dominance (the functional differences between homologous areas of the two hemispheres of the brain), and the relationship of cerebral pathology to impairments of language processes.

The contents of this chapter are not in any way to be considered as definitive treatment or as a substitute for several excellent detailed considerations of the subject. The materials have been selected in the hope that they will provide the reader with the bases for understanding

Chapter 3

what brain mechanisms may be impaired in the special population of children who fail to acquire language, or who are seriously delayed in this acquisition, although they are neither mentally retarded nor severely impaired in hearing. Extended considerations of brain mechanisms and language functioning may be found in the writings of Penfield and Roberts (1959), Schuell, Jenkins, and Jimenez-Pabon (1964), Luria (1966), and Millikan and Darley (1967). Briefer and more specialized discussions may be found in Masland (1967, 1968), Geschwind (1964), Lenneberg (1967), and Eisenson, Auer, and Irwin (1963).

We will begin our consideration of the brain mechanisms that underlie language functioning (speech) by a brief description of the structure of the cerebrum.

The Cerebrum (Brain)

The cerebrum consists of two apparently symmetrical, almost mirror-image hemispheres. The outer surface of the cerebrum is a thin layer of gray matter, which contains cell bodies. Beneath the gray surface is a thick layer of white matter consisting largely of fibers covered by myelin (white nerve sheathing). These fibers run to and from the cells of the cortex. The interior of the cerebrum consists of four cavities or ventricles.

The Cerebral Cortex

The cerebral cortex is the gray outer layer of the cerebrum. It is characterized by its many folds or indentations. The nature of this construction provides additional surface for the gray matter and for the ten to twelve billion or more of nerve cells to carry out their complex functions related to the reception, integration, and interpretation of stimuli and to the organization and expression of human behavior. Our special interest will be for that form of human species–specific behavior we refer to as speech.

The shallow indentations or furrows of the cortex are known as *sulci* (singular, sulcus). The deeper indentations are known as *fissures*. The fissures permit us to consider the cortex as "divided" into major regions or lobes: the frontal (anterior), the temporal, the occipital (posterior), and the parietal. Another major area, the *insula*, or Island of Reil, is within the lateral fissure and is, therefore, not visible on the surface of the cortex.

Functional Areas

The cortex in broad plan may be considered to have two kinds of specialized centers or regions: projection and association areas. Those parts of the cortex that receive or send nerve fibers to or from the peripheral organs of the body are known as *projection areas*. These may be defined as regions of the cortex that communicate with lower centers of the central nervous system through specific nerve tracts. In addition, the cerebral cortex also contains association areas, which lie adjacent to the projection areas. Association areas make connections only with other regions of the cortex. Functionally, association areas may be considered as regions of the cortex that integrate nerve impulses, which are received from projection areas. Association areas are for the most part considerably larger than the projection areas. In the anterior and posterior parts of the cerebrum, the frontal and occipital lobes, the association areas are particularly large. It is assumed that the interrelationships between the activities of the sensory and motor areas take place in the association cortex. Thus, presumably, complex functions such as listening and speaking are able to be integrated and produced. Figure 1 features some of the projection and association areas that have special significance for speech (language) functions.

The Thalamus and Striate Bodies

The *thalamus* is a mass of cerebral tissue which is situated at the base of the cerebrum and projects into the third ventricle of the brain. The thalamus is relay station for sensory (incoming) stimuli. All auditory, visual, visceral, and somatic stimuli either terminate in the thalamus or make connections there which continue on to the projection areas of the cerebral cortex.

The *striate bodies* are three gray nuclear masses which lie beneath the white matter in the forepart of the cerebral cortex. The nerve pathways that go to and from the cortex pass through the striate bodies. Functionally, in regard to speech, the striate bodies may be considered as a unit of the thalamus.

The Hypothalamus

The hypothalamus is located directly beneath the thalamus. Modifications in the control of the visceral organs associated with

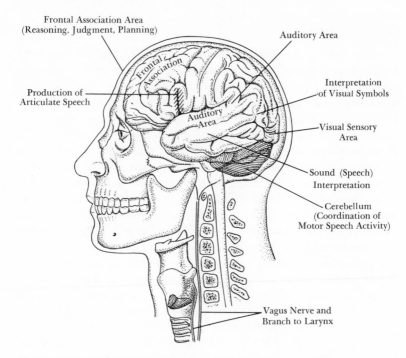

Figure 1. Localization of brain function in relation to speech.

emotional responses, e.g., changes in heart rate and blood pressure, are a result of activities of centers in the hypothalamus.

The Cerebellum

The cerebellum or small brain is situated directly below the cerebrum and partly covered by it. The cerebellum has many complex connections throughout the entire nervous system. It has sensory connections with the nerve fibers that convey proprioceptive (muscle) sensitivity from the muscles of the body and from the balance mechanism of the inner ear. Coordination and control of voluntary movements are made possible by the elaborate connections between the cerebellum and the cerebrum. Presumably also, precision of timing (synergy of movement) and the general character and tonus of muscular responses, both reflex and voluntary, take place as a result of the controls "imposed" by the cerebellum.

Probably the best example of this function is the finely timed and coordinated motor activities involved in an act of speech.

The Brain Stem

The cerebrum and cerebellum are connected by large columns of neural tissue and central masses which are part of the brain stem. The lower (posterior) part of the brain stem is a flattened, cone-shaped mass known as the *medulla oblongata*. This part of the brain stem is, by way of an opening in the base of the skull, continuous with the spinal cord. The anterior part of the brain stem, which includes the thalamus, is continuous with the cerebrum. Later we shall discuss the reticular formation, which for the most part consists of a neural network in the brain stem.

The Midbrain

The midbrain lies immediately below the thalamus. By means of connections with the cerebellum and the medulla, the midbrain has essential functions related to the regulation of muscle tone, body posture, and movement. By way of other centers, the midbrain is involved with functions that are integrated in the cerebral hemispheres. Of particular importance are reflexes controlling the eye.

The Pons

The pons is a unit of the central nervous system that lies just below the midbrain. This area, as the name suggests, serves as a bridge between the two sides of the cerebellum. Neural pathways to and from the cerebellum merge in the area of the pons.

The Medulla Oblongata

The medulla, or bulb, as we indicated earlier, is a flattened cone-shaped mass continuous with the brain stem and spinal cord. Nerve tracts (pyramidal tracts) come to the medulla from the cerebral cortex. These tracts cross over (decussate) at the narrower, posterior end of the medulla. The medulla also has sensory tracts going toward the higher centers. In addition, the medulla has

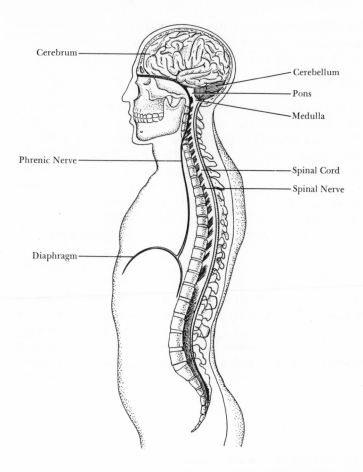

Cerebrum

Cerebellum

Pons

Medulla

Phrenic Nerve

Spinal Cord

Spinal Nerve

Diaphragm

Figure 2. The central nervous system in relation to speech. The cerebrum: normal meaningful speech is dependent upon the integrative activity of the parts of the cerebrum. The cerebellum "sorts and arranges" muscular impulses that come to it from higher brain centers. Impulses are here correlated so that precise muscular activity such as is needed for speech becomes possible. The pons is a bridge of nerve fibers between the cerebral cortex and the medulla. The medulla contains the respiratory and other reflex centers. The spinal cord and its nerves control the respiratory muscles. The phrenic nerve emerges from the spinal cord in the neck region and extends to the diaphragm. It supplies the impulses that cause the diaphragm to contract in breathing. (From Eisenson, J., and Boase, P. H., *Basic Speech,* New York, Macmillan, 1964, p. 28.)

centers that are vital to biological functioning. These include the functions of respiration and circulation.

The spinal cord is continuous with the lower (posterior) portion of the medulla. Nerves emanating from the spinal cord go to the peripheral organs of the body.

Figure 2 is a diagrammatic representation of the central nervous system in relation to speech.

The Reticular Formation

The reticular formation is a rather vaguely defined organization or system of nerve cells in the brain stem. The cells of the reticular formation include fibers that extend (project) to the spinal cord, the cerebellum, and the cerebral hemispheres. In turn, the reticular formation also receives fibers from the same structures. Thus, the reticular formation may be functionally considered to have *ascending* and *descending* parts.

The ascending part of the reticular system seems, in effect, to constitute a "central station" where nerve impulses arrive from the receptor organs—the ears, eyes, nose, and the skin. Impulses from the reticular central station are conducted to various parts of the brain, including the projection centers of the cerebral cortex.

The *descending* reticular formation receives impulses from the cerebral cortex and, in turn, sends impulses to the numerous fibers that come to it from the receptor organs. In this way, presumably, neural signals coming down from the cortex meet signals coming up from the receptors. As a result, there is a selection of responses that may be made (perceptual selection). As an example, according to Krech and Crutchfield (1958 p. 172):

. . . an impulse that comes down from the occipital lobe of the brain (the visual center) through the descending reticular formation can prevent impulses coming up from the ear from ever reaching the cortex. This can help us to understand the very common experience of not hearing someone speak to us when all our attention is directed at watching an object intently.

Although there is as yet no general agreement as to all the possible functions of the reticular formation, there is agreement that one of its very important functions is to maintain a state of consciousness (awareness and alertness). Thus, we may generalize

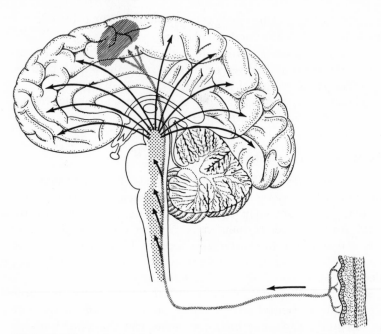

Figure 3. The reticular formation is the stippled area in this cross section of the brain. A sense organ (lower right) is connected to a sensory area in the brain (upper left) by a pathway extending up the spinal cord. This pathway branches into the reticular formation. When a stimulus travels along the pathway, the reticular formation may "awaken" the entire brain (dark arrows). (From French, J. D., "The Reticular Formation." Copyright © (1957) by *Scientific American, Inc.* All rights reserved.)

to the effect that nerve impulses from the ascending part of the reticular formation serve to arouse or alert the cortex so that normal perception may take place. So, according to Penfield and Roberts (1959, p. 16), the reticular system "provides neuronal mechanisms which seem to be essential to consciousness and the integration of function in the cerebral hemispheres." Lindsley (1961) indicates that in addition to serving as an arousal mechanism, the reticular formation may also serve as a specific attention mechanism, thus permitting the individual to make the appropriate differential responses (perceptual integration) to environmental stimuli. A third function served by the reticular formation is that of a feedback-control mechanism.

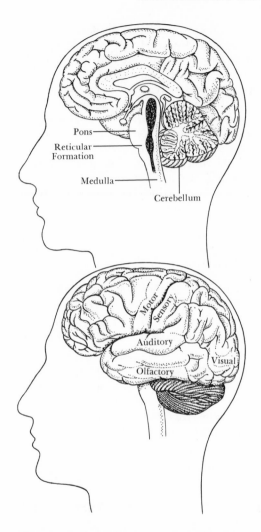

Figure 4. Relationship of the reticular formation (black area) to various parts of the brain is indicated at the top. The functional areas of the brain are outlined at bottom. (From French, J. D., "The Reticular Formation." Copyright © (1957) by *Scientific American, Inc.* All rights reserved.)

We may summarize some of the contributions of the reticular formation to cerebral functioning in particular and to human behavior in general by a citation from French (1957):

The reticular formation is a tiny nerve network in the central part of the brain stem. Investigators have discovered that this bit of nerve tissue, no bigger than your little finger, is a far more important structure than anyone has dreamed. It underlies our awareness of the world and our ability to think, to learn and to act. Without it an individual is reduced to a helpless, senseless, paralyzed blob of protoplasm.

The actual seat of the power to think, to perceive, indeed to respond to a stimulus with anything more than a reflex reaction, lies in the cortex of the brain. But the cortex cannot perceive or think unless it is "awake." . . . A sensory signal arriving at the cortex while it is asleep goes unrecognized. Experiments on anesthetized individuals have shown . . . that stimulation of the cortex alone is not sufficient to awaken the brain. Something else must arouse the cortex: that something else is the reticular formation.

Contralaterality of Cerebral Control

In our discussion of the medulla we indicated that nerve tracts come to the medulla from the cortex and cross over (decussate) in the lower portion. This is an example of the general plan of the nervous system, which results in contralateral control of motor and sensory functions. Thus, movements of the organs on the right side of the body are controlled by centers of the motor tract of the left cerebral hemisphere. Sensory function for paired receptors, the eyes and the ears, present a somewhat different arrangement. There are some fibers that do not cross. However, as we will note from our diagrammatic representation for the ears (Figure 5), the greater number of fibers do cross, so that the basic scheme of contralaterality of the higher brain functions is maintained.

Cerebral Dominance and Differences in Cerebral Functions

In our description of the cerebrum we referred to it as consisting of two symmetrical, almost mirror-image hemispheres. Despite the physical similarity of the hemispheres, functionally there are important differences (Eisenson, 1971).[1]

[1]It is important to appreciate that the two hemispheres of the brain are not really as alike as superficially they appear to be. Geschwind and Levitsky (1968) "have found marked anatomical asymmetries between the upper surfaces of the human right and left temporal lobes." The area is significantly larger on the left side and ". . . the differences observed are easily of sufficient magnitude to be compatible with the known functional asymmetries."

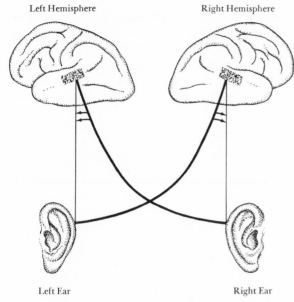

Figure 5. Neuroanatomical schema for auditory asymmetries indicating crossing of nerve fibers. (After Kimura, D., "Functional Asymmetry of the Brain in Dichotic Listening," *Cortex, 3,* 2, 1967, p. 174.)

Some of the differences, based on clinical evidence following pathology, include the following:

1. The perception of spatial events (spatial perception, awareness of body scheme, and spatial relationships) are predominantly a function of centers in the right hemisphere (Masland, 1967, pp. 17–19).

2. The perception of auditory, nonspeech events (environmental noises, musical melody, tonal patterns, etc.) is processed (controlled) in the right hemisphere.

3. The perception of speech events is normally a function of the left hemisphere, and specifically of centers of the left temporal lobe.[2]

From what we have just indicated in regard to differences in cerebral functioning, the question of cerebral dominance or cere-

[2]These observations and others in relationship to differences in cerebral functioning are considered in detail in Mountcastle (1962) and Millikan and Darley (1967).

bral control is related to function. Some functions are dominated or controlled by the left hemisphere, others by the right. Language functions, the perception of the symbols of speech and of writing, and the production of spoken and written language are controlled (dominated) by centers of the left cerebral hemisphere for 95 percent or more of right-handed persons and for a majority of left-handed persons.

The Left Brain Is for Talking

As we indicated above, recent findings on the differences between the two hemispheres permit us to generalize that normally the left brain is for talking. Primarily, this is so because the left cerebral hemisphere, and particularly the left temporal lobe, is the processor of speech signals. Speech is normally established through listening. Thus, we accept the conclusions of Liberman *et al.* (1967) that "the conclusion that there is a speech mode, and that it is characterized by processes different from those underlying the perception of other sounds, is strengthened by recent indications that speech and non-speech sounds are processed primarily in different hemispheres of the brain."

Although human beings are born with the potential for differential hearing (listening), the differences do not seem to become clearly established until about age four or five, and usually somewhat earlier for girls than for boys (Kimura, 1967). It is of interest that Kimura reports that children from low socioeconomic groups in Montreal, Canada, appear to be later in this functional development than do children from high socioeconomic groups. Further, Kimura found that children with reading problems, especially boys, show a lag in this development.[3]

Laterality and Cerebral Dominance

Except for a small percentage of the ambidextrous and the ambi-nondextrous, most children establish hand preference by age five. Along with these preferences most children also establish eyedness and footedness. Perhaps about 20 percent of us have mixed laterality preference, so that some of us may be right-handed

[3]Kimura's investigations were based on the expression of ear preference, which is believed to be related to cerebral dominance. We shall discuss ear preference later. For an exposition of Kimura's investigations see Kimura (1967).

and left-eyed, or left-handed and right-eyed. Laterality preference in general, and handedness in particular, may be a result of several factors. Propably chief of these factors is hereditary or constitutional predisposition. However, environmental pressures may induce a potentially left-handed child to learn to use his right hand for writing and possibly for eating. Injury to a hand or arm may cause a change from inclined or established handedness. Psychological factors such as identification may exert influence in handedness. Negativism may exert a contrary influence. Early brain pathology may limit laterality expression, and later brain damage may leave no choice except to make a change. Normally, however, once handedness is established, it tends to be maintained for life. Although, as we have indicated, handedness is only one form of laterality, it is probably the best single indicator of overall laterality preference.

Ear Preference

Unless an individual has a serious hearing impairment of one ear, he of course listens with both ears. Normally, our ears listen together rather than competitively. Normally also, if the occasion arises for listening with one ear, as we do in most telephone situations, or when someone whispers into an ear, either ear can do alone what both ears usually do together. However, suppose we were required to listen competitively, that is, to have different signals sent simultaneously, one signal or series of signals to one ear, and a different signal or series of signals sent to the other, how would the signals be heard? Would there be an indication of ear preference, and if so, would such preference be related to other aspects of laterality expression, and especially to handedness? The answer, based on recent experimental investigations, seems to be positive. Some of the investigations, which are reviewed by Kimura (1967), employ the technique of dichotic (competitive) listening devised by Broadbent (1954). The basic technique sets up competition between the two ears for the reception of auditory signals. In the initial Broadbent study, different digits were presented simultaneously to a listener's ears by means of a dual-channel tape recorder with stereophonic earphones. One sequence of digits was presented to one ear while another sequence was simultaneously (competitively) presented to the other ear. The subject was asked to report all the digits he could recall in whatever order he could recall them. Because the investigator knew the ear to which the digit sequences were sent, the report of the subject provided separate scores for the recall ability of each ear. The usual finding for normal right-handed persons is a statistically significant greater recall for those digits that were sent to the right ear than for those sent to the left. We can report that investigations using speech signals other than digits, e.g., words or short verbal utterances (Dirks, 1964), show results along the same lines as those found by Broadbent. In interesting contrast are findings when melodies rather than speech signals are presented to subjects dichotically. In such a study Kimura (1967) found that nonverbal, melodic material is recognized more accurately by the left ear than by the right. Thus, we may conclude that ear preferences are part of overall laterality preference. The dichotic listening investigations provide support for the observation made earlier that there is a speech mode, and that the processing of speech is different from the processing of nonspeech auditory events. We emphasize this point because it sheds light on the clinical observation that most congenitally aphasic children can respond appropriately to environmental noises other than speech long before they can understand and respond to speech.

Although ear preference and hand preference are both normally established by age four or five, we do not wish to suggest that the two are in any way causally related. Neither do we wish in any way to leave an impression that left-handed persons have left ear preference. In fact, most left-handed persons show the same preference, though not to the same degree, for speech and nonspeech, as do right-handed persons. To return to an earlier statement, the left hemisphere is for speaking, for the perception, control, and production of speech—for almost all right-handed persons as well as for a majority of those who are left-handed. Similarly, the right cerebral hemisphere, regardless of handedness, seems to be dominant for environmental, nonspeech auditory events.

Localization of Language Functions

As we suggested earlier, most of what we know about the brain mechanisms that serve or control language functions is based on information from the pathology of impairment. Human brains have been "mapped" for lesions that are associated with disruptions of language functions which were established before the pathology was incurred. Based on such knowledge it is assumed that certain areas of the cerebral cortex are normally in control of particular language functions; that is, the areas make special contribution to cerebral functioning as a whole, in regard to language (speech). Figure 1 diagrams the left cerebral cortex featuring the major areas whose function underlies the normal acquisition of language.[4]

Based on data from several sources (Penfield and Roberts, 1959; Russell and Esper, 1961; Luria, 1965; and from Masland's research review articles, 1967 and 1968) and from the evidence presented in our earlier discussion, the following general observations may be made:

1. The left cerebral hemisphere serves overall language functions for a vast majority of persons, regardless of individual handedness.

2. Productive language functions are served by the anterior portions of the cerebral cortex.

3. Receptive or intake functions (the decoding of language) are served by the posterior portions. Auditory decoding is carried on in the left temporal area, and visual decoding primarily in the left occipital lobe.

The Auditory Cortex

We have made several references to the left temporal lobe and its functions, which are related to the perception of spoken language. Earlier we also cited the article by Geschwind and Levitsky (1968) who report anatomical differences between the left and right temporal areas "of sufficient magnitude to be compatible with the known functional asymmetries." We will now expand on the particular functions of the temporal lobe that are fundamental for the perception of the speech code.

Speech, as we point out in our discussion in the chapter on perception, is a sequential or time-bound, function. We also pointed out that temporal-order resolution is impaired in aphasic adults and seems to be impaired or slow in development in aphasic

---

[4]The evidence of the investigations of dichotic listening referred to earlier permits us to make observations relative to auditory functioning of normal persons as well as to the effects of pathology. The findings on normal persons support the evidence coming from those following pathology.

children. Hearing and language, as Masland notes (see Millikan and Darley, 1967, p. 234), require a preoccupation with time or temporal order. In listening to speech the hearer must make continuous and very rapid decisions about sequential auditory events. Thus, Masland says, "I have been intrigued with the possibility that maybe it is the integration of time bound activities which centers in the left hemisphere. . . ." We believe this to be so. Further, it appears that time-bound activities are impaired in the event of damage to the left temporal lobe.

Speech-sound (phonemic) discrimination is also served by the left temporal area. The effect of lesion on phonemic perception may be appreciated from the data of Figure 6.

On the positive side Luria (1966, p. 101) indicates that the essential function of the left temporal lobe (the secondary divisions of the auditory cortex of the left hemisphere) is in

The analysis and integration of the sound flow by identification of the phonemic signs of the objective system of the language. This work must be carried out with the very close participation of articulatory acts which . . . constitute the efferent link for the perception of the sounds of speech. It consists of differentiating the significant, phonemic signs of the spoken sounds, inhibiting the unessential signs, and comparing the perceived sound complexes on this phonemic basis.

An inspection of the diagram for localization of function in relationship to speech (Figure 1) will reveal the close proximity of the area for the control of articulate speech to the auditory cortex. We also suggest a review of our basic definition of perception in relationship to Luria's emphasis that the auditory cortex differentiates the significant phonemic signs of speech signals and compares "the perceived sound complexes on this phonemic basis."

Exceptions to Left Cerebral Control

Although the left cerebral hemisphere is normally dominant for language function, there are some important exceptions. These exceptions include a very small minority of right-handed persons and perhaps a bare majority of natural left-handed persons. The latter group, based on their ability for spontaneous recovery of language following acquired damage to the left hemisphere, seem to have either (a) bilateral cerebral control for language, or (b) in the event of damage to the left hemisphere, a capacity for the right hemisphere to assume controls normally served by the left.

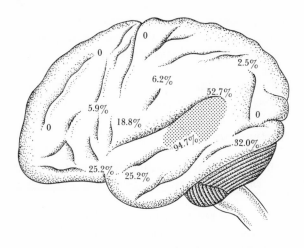

Figure 6. Percentage distribution of cases with impaired phonemic perception related to site of cerebral lesion. Stipple region includes the auditory projection and association areas considered to be essential for normal phonemic perception. Note the relatively high incidence of impaired phonemic perception related to lesions in areas immediately adjacent to the stippled region. (After Masland, R. L., "Some Neurological Processes Underlying Language," *Annals of Otology, Rhinology,* and *Laryngology,* 77, 4, 1968, 787; based on data from Luria, A. R., "Brain Disorders and Language Analysis," *Language and Speech,* 1, 1, 1958, 14–34.)

Another important exceptional group is found in young persons, below age twelve, who also make excellent recovery of language function in the event of acquired damage to the left hemisphere. In this group we may assume that the plasticity of the young brain is such as to make a shift in cerebral dominance for language which is not ordinarily the case in older persons (Penfield and Roberts, 1959, p. 102; Penfield, 1971).

From our brief review of cerebral dominance and language function, it is evident that though the left cerebral cortex is normally dominant (normally subserves language), the right hemisphere has the capability or potentiality for subserving language under certain conditions. One of these conditions, pointed out by Masland (1967), is found in children who incur serious injury to the brain and in children whose entire left hemispheres are removed prior to approximately eight years of age. Most of these children, after recovery from the physical effects of the operation, resume language functions and seem to be able to talk normally. The assumption is that these children reestablished language function under the control of the right cerebral hemisphere. Masland raises the question: "If that is the case, what is the basis of the language disability of those children who *do* have language disabilities?" He offers several possible explanations:

1. These children suffer from bilateral lesions involving both hemispheres.

2. The defect (lesion) lies in lower centers (the brain stem or basal ganglia) through which information is relayed to the higher brain structures.

3. "There are genetically or constitutionally determined organizational defects or peculiarities of the brain of such individuals which cause it to be difficult or impossible for them to form the associations or correlations essential to the establishment of language" (Masland, 1967).

A fourth possibility which we considered in our discussion on perceptual dysfunction is the position of Eisenberg (1964, pp. 68–69) who notes:

The psychological deficits we observe in the patient who has suffered early cerebral injury cannot be taken to imply that the tissue destroyed is in itself the sole cause of the entire pattern. The injury might have impaired an elementary psychological function, the lack of which could then distort subsequent development. Thus, complex functions, the anatomical equipment for which might otherwise be intact, could have failed to evolve.

We believe that the same effects of psychological dysfunction, which Eisenberg suggests may come from brain lesion, might also be a result of maturational delay.

REFERENCES

Broadbent, D. E., "The Role of Auditory Localization in Attention and Memory Span," *Journal of Experimental Psychology,* 1954, 47, 191–196.

Dirks, D., "Perception of Dichotic and Monaural Verbal Material and Cerebral Dominance for Speech," *Acta Otololaryngologia,* 58, 1964, 73–80.

Eisenberg, L., "Behavioral Manifestations of Cerebral Damage in Childhood," in *Brain Damage in Children,* Birch, H. G., ed., Baltimore, Williams and Wilkins, 1964.

Eisenson, J., "The Left Brain is for Talking," *Acta Symbolica,* 2, 1, 1971, 33–36.

———, Auer, J. J., and Irwin, J. V., *Psychology of Communication,* New York, Appleton-Century-Crofts, 1963, chap. 4.

French, J. D., "The Reticular Formation," *Scientific America,* 196, 5, 1957, 54–60.

Geschwind, N., "The Development of the Brain and the Evolution of Language," *Monograph Series on Language and Linguistics,* no. 17, 1964, 155–169.

Geschwind, A. N., and Levitsky, W., "Human Brain: Left-Right Asymmetries in Temporal Speech Region," *Science,* 161, 1968, 186–187.

Kimura, D., "Functional Asymmetry of the Brain in Dichotic Listening," *Cortex,* 3, 1967, 163–178.

Krech, D., and Crutchfield, R. S., *Elements of Psychology,* New York, Knopf, 1958.

Lenneberg, E. H., *Biological Foundations of Language,* New York, Wiley, 1967, 52–76.

Liberman, A. M., Cooper, F. S., Shankweiler, D. P., and Studdert-Kennedy, M., "Perception of the Speech Code," *Psychological Review,* 74, 6, 1967, 431–461.

Lindsley, D. B., "The Reticular Activation System and Perceptual Integration," in *Electrical Stimulation of the Brain,* Sheer, D. E., ed., Austin, University of Texas Press, 1961, 331–349.

Luria, A. R., *Higher Cortical Functions in Man,* New York, Basic Books, 1966.

———, "Aspects of Aphasia," *Journal of the Neurological Sciences,* 2, 3, 1965, 278–287.

Masland, R. L., "Some Neurological Processes Underlying Language," *Annals of Otology, Rhinology and Laryngology,* 77, 4, 1968, 787.

———, "Brain Mechanisms Underlying the Language Function," *Bulletin of the Orton Society,* 1967, 17, 1, 1–31.

Millikan, C. H., and Darley, F. L., eds., *Brain Mechanisms Underlying Speech and Language,* New York, Grune and Stratton, 1967.

Mountcastle, V. B., ed., *Interhemispheric Relations and Cerebral Dominance,* Baltimore, Johns Hopkins Press, 1962.

Penfield, W., "Language Learning and the 'Switch Mechanism,'" *Acta Symbolica,* 2, 1, 1971, 22–32.

———, and Roberts, L., *Speech and Brain Mechanisms,* Princeton, N.J., Princeton University Press, 1959.

Russell, W. R., and Espir, M. L. E., *Traumatic Aphasia,* London, Oxford University Press, 1961.

Schuell, H., Jenkins, J. J., and Jimenez-Pabon, E., *Aphasia in Adults,* New York, Harper and Row, 1964, chap. 4.

Developmental Aphasia [Dyslogia]

We will state with emphasis at the outset that the severely developmentally aphasic (dyslogic) child is a rare child indeed. However rare, he does exist and is a puzzle to himself, a source and cause of bewilderment to his parents, and a challenge to the pediatrician, educator, psychologist, and language clinician for understanding, diagnosis, and appropriate treatment.

Some authorities on language disorders take exception to the use of the term *aphasia* as a designation for failure or delayed language development in a child even when there is positive evidence of neurological damage. The argument is along purist, semantic lines. *Aphasia,* which literally means without speech but which has come to mean

Chapter 4

severe impairment of previously established language functions, is therefore necessarily an acquired rather than congenital or developmental involvement (Critchley, 1967, pp. 3–25). In another publication (Eisenson and Ogilvie, 1971, chap. 16) we introduced the term *dyslogia* to designate the child who though not deaf, nor mentally retarded, nor autistic, nevertheless presents evidence of central nervous system involvement associated with severe language delay. The neurological involvements sometimes include "hard" signs. More often, "soft" signs, such as those usually associated with *minimal brain dysfunction,* are found. However, since man has a way with words that sometimes defies rules of logic and semantics, the terms *aphasia, dysphasia,* and *aphasoid* continue to be used in the current literature to designate the dyslogic (nonverbal) child. So we shall in our discussion use the term *dyslogia* and *dyslogic* as synonymous with *developmental* or *congenital aphasia* and *aphasic.* However, a child who has acquired language and subsequently has suffered impairment as a result of cerebral damage through accident or disease is an aphasic child without the need for a modifying adjective. Fortunately, because of the plasticity of the young brain, almost all young aphasic children—up to age twelve or so—make remarkably good recoveries from these acquired impairments. The exceptions are found among those children who incur bilateral and diffuse cerebral damage. Why a child with congenital unilateral cerebral damage has great difficulty in acquiring language whereas one who has incurred comparable damage, at least comparable as far as our present assessment procedures can determine, can usually quickly and spontaneously reestablish language remains one of the great mysteries of human neuropathology.

The Syndrome of Developmental Aphasia (Dyslogia)

Children who are born with brain damage because of a prenatal (congenital) condition, or who are markedly delayed in cerebral maturation, or who incurred brain damage before the onset of speech, are frequently severely retarded in language development. Some of these children are frankly cerebral palsied as well as aphasic. Others, especially those who have bilateral cerebral damage, may also be mentally retarded. A few may have severe hearing impairment. Our present considerations will be limited to these low incidence but fascinating children who are (a) *not* mentally retarded, but who may have learning impairments to suggest otherwise, (b) who are not deaf or even moderately hard of hearing, but in some ways suggest that they might be so, and (c) who are not severely autistic (nonrelating to human beings and so possibly nonspeaking), but who all too often withdraw from human speakers because of their inability to make sense out of human (speech) sounds.

Some children who may be initially developmentally aphasic on the basis of slow maturation of their central nervous systems may have delayed onset of speech and be slower than expected in their speech development. They may, at age four or five, present a profile in language development in many ways comparable to that of a two-year-old. We have found this so in our investigations at the Institute for Childhood Aphasia at Stanford University. Some children are slow in their phonemic (articulatory) development, have a limited vocabulary that is suggestive of a child who is just beginning to speak, and retarded syntactic proficiency. Their overall profile shadows, but does not quite parallel that of younger normal-speaking children. Other children, however, present diverse and scattered language profiles, so that we are not yet ready to generalize that a developmentally aphasic child is a retarded shadow of his age peer.

Differential Diagnostic Features of Developmental Aphasia

As we indicated earlier, the developmentally aphasic (dyslogic) child often behaves as if he is mentally retarded, or has a profound hearing loss, or is autistic. Therefore, our differential diagnostic criteria must serve to distinguish him from other language-delayed and nonverbal children. Differential features include the following:[1]

1. Perceptual dysfunctions are in one or more sensory modalities, but not in all modalities. Auditory perception is almost invariably involved. By perception we mean the process by which an individual organizes received sensory data, compares this organized input with other input stored in his memory, and assigns meaning on some category or level to the new input. Thus, we may

[1]For detailed considerations see Eisenson, "Developmental Aphasia: A Speculative View with Therapeutic Considerations" (1968); Eisenson, "Developmental Patterns of Non-Verbal Children" (1966); and Eisenson and Ogilvie (1971), chap. 16.

say that the individual has received and decoded input. Essentially, then, the process of perception implies an act of categorization according to which the individual receives sensory stimulation and responds by identifying, sorting, and giving meaning to it. Usually, but not necessarily, the individual gives expression to his intake by an *appropriate form of output*. When this does take place, we may use the hyphenated term perceptual-motor response (Kephart, 1960, p. 63; Eisenson, 1966b).

2. Auditory dysfunction is in excess of what would ordinarily be implied on the basis of conventionally determined (audiometric) hearing loss. Such dysfunction includes difficulty in speech sound (phonemic) discrimination and phonemic sequencing. By sequencing we mean the capacity to hold a series of events in mind and to respond to an ongoing event in the light of immediately past events. Because speech is a flow of sounds, a child who can discriminate but cannot sequence the flow or stream of auditory events will not be able to understand what he hears. He may, in effect, be able to hear but not to "aud" or listen to speech (Hardy, 1962).

3. Sequencing difficulties are pronounced for auditory events and especially for speech, but may also be present for visual events.

4. Intellectual inefficiency is over and above any objectively determined mental limitation. Since we are working on the assumption that we are dealing with children who are not mentally retarded, we are implying that they may not have functional intelligence consistent with expectations based on their mental age and their intelligence quotients. Observation indicates that the developmentally aphasic child requires optimal conditions— an absence of distraction and of "noise" of any variety to function up to his intellectual potential even in situations where language processing is not involved. A little bit of distraction, or of fatigue, or of awareness of error may go a long way to impair the intellectual functioning of the aphasic child. In this sense, we regard him as being intellectually inefficient.

If we observe an aphasic child's test performance or performance in a learning situation, we may note considerable variability on the same type of task or test from time to time during a day, as well as from day to day. If we accept the child's best performance as indicative of his intellectual potential, then developmentally aphasic children tend to approximate the norm in intellectual functioning, at least when the assessment is made on the basis of nonverbal standardized test inventories.

Dr. Joel Stark, while a member of the Institute for Childhood Aphasia at Stanford University, studied the test performance of 75 aphasic children ranging from three through eight years of age. He employed two scales, the Leiter International (Arthur adaptation) and the Columbia Mental Maturity, both of which can be administered without verbal directions and which require no verbal responses. The final diagnosis for the children in the Stark study was severe language impairment associated with established or likely CNS involvement. The results are summarized in Table 2.

TABLE 2. Test Scores of 75 Aphasic Children, Age Range 3–8 Years; Columbia Mental Maturity Scale (CMMS) and the Leiter International Performance Scale (LIPS)

		CMMS		LIPS	
Age Group	N	Mean IQ	SD	Mean IQ	SD
3–4.11	16	99.5	17.95	93.8	22.18
5–6.11	35	87.0	12.59	89.3	21.06
7–8.11	24	73.1	16.56	79.4	12.62

We may note that the mean IQ for the three- and four-year-old children is normal. Also to be noted is the lower-than-average IQ for the older children. We interpret this difference in scores to be a reflection of the difference in task requirements related to form, color, and size. At the upper age level correct performance requires an ability to categorize and abstract, and either to select an item on the Columbia or to arrange materials on the Leiter, according to some principle. An additional factor in the upper-level items is that each test situation involves the child in having to deal with considerably more stimuli than at the lower levels.

Observations of the behavior of the children when they are confronted with difficult items reveal a marked tendency to perseveration, displays of anger and hostility directed either at the materials or the test administrator, and often considerable hyperactivity. Some children, however, simply withdraw from further involvement with the testing situation. Another clinical observation of the test performance of these children is their inclination to lose sight of the principle necessary for the completion of a task. For example, if a test task calls for the alternation of figures, such as a circle and a square, a child may arrange half of the number of figures in the appropriate order, and then place the others in a completely random order. Another characteristic performance error is the failure to carry over a principle from one test task to another. Thus, if, as on the Columbia scale, a child succeeds in pointing to the appropriate (different) figure, we still cannot assume that he will remember the principle of this task for succeeding items. His performance may improve if he is reminded of the nature of the task for each succeeding item. This is ordinarily not required for normal children.

5. Language development may be so retarded that the child at age four or five may still be essentially nonverbal both for the comprehension and production of speech. In other instances as we indicated earlier, the child may have had a delayed onset of speech, perhaps with first words between 24 and 30 months, and at age four or older be at a two-word phrase level when most of their age peers are using conventional syntax. In general we may describe the productive language of the less severely impaired developmentally aphasic child as being sparse in vocabulary and lacking in syntactic competence. As we indicated earlier, he may shadow the linguistic proficiencies of his age peers.

A-phasic Development of the Congenitally Aphasic Child

By hyphenating a-phasic we are directing attention to the out-of-phase developmental background of congenitally aphasic children. Clinical histories reveal that these children often do not present the anticipated patterns and correlations of their age peers in regard to their general sensory, motor, and perceptual abilities as well as in their intellectual abilities. Even when brain dysfunction cannot be established on a hard-sign basis, the congenitally aphasic child indicates by his clinical history that he is *brain different*. Morley (1960) reported similar findings in a longitudinal study of aphasic children. Aphasic children are slow to develop laterality for handedness and, we believe, for the establishment of ear preference.

Neurological Findings

As we have indicated, many developmentally aphasic children do not present clear-cut or hard-sign evidence of central nervous system pathology. Perhaps about one child in two or three, who on the basis of psychological and psycholinguistic assessment is designated as an aphasic child, also shows clear evidence of neuropathology. Many more, at least another third, show evidence "of at least minimal brain damage" (Brown, 1967, p. 357), or minimal brain dysfunction. Perhaps it is more accurate to suggest that these children show evidence of maximum brain dysfunction despite minimal evidence of brain damage.

Electroencephalographic (EEG) Findings

Several investigations indicate that abnormal EEG findings occur in a higher incidence among congenitally aphasic children than we expect from children in their age range who are not aphasic. Goldstein, Landau, and Kleffner (1958) report that about 40 percent of 69 aphasic children showed abnormal EEG findings. This percentage was about the same as for 114 deaf children with whom those with aphasia were compared. However, the aphasic children had a higher incidence of focal abnormalities (14.5 percent compared with 6.1 percent for the deaf). In a study at the Institute for Childhood Aphasia at Stanford University, about half (36 of 73) aphasic children had abnormal EEG's. Twenty-two of the abnormalities were localized, of which nineteen were in the left cerebral hemisphere. This, perhaps, is the most significant part of the observations because, as we have indicated, the left cerebral hemisphere is the one normally assumed to be dominant for speech.

Phonemic or Speech-Sound Imperception

Now let us return to the implications of some of our neurologic findings for the understanding of the developmentally aphasic child's difficulty with normal speech perception and, therefore, for the acquisition of speech. With only rare exception we consider the aphasic child's basic perceptual impairment to be one for auditory perception for speech at the rate at which speech is normally presented. Even though some aphasic children may have a mild hearing loss and a few a moderate loss based on audiometric results, the typical pure-tone audiogram would be such as to be described as adequate for speech. For the developmentally aphasic child, the correlation between audiometric findings and hearing (really *listening*) for speech does not pertain. Even if a speech threshold is established to suggest that the child "hears" speech at a given level, which is presumably low enough so that he should be able to learn to speak, other factors prevent or delay this acquisition. The most important of these factors is difficulty in speech-sound or phonemic discrimination in contextual utterance.

Luria, the Russian neuropsychologist (1966, pp. 106–107), holds that an area of the left temporal cortex, which he designates as the *auditory cortex*, has a special capacity for phonemic (speech-sound) discrimination. Thus, delayed maturation or damage to this area is likely to result in impairment for speech-sound discrimination and perception. However, we should note that appropriate perception of nonspeech environmental sounds may not be impaired. This probably accounts for the apparent inconsistency of the developmentally aphasic child's responses to sounds that are appropriate to animal, mechanical, and other environmental noises, but inappropriate to speech. Perhaps the developmentally aphasic child is not really as inconsistent a listener as he superficially appears to be. Those of us who logically expect that a child who is able to hear and understand environmental sounds should also be able to hear and understand all sounds, including speech, may well be the ones who are in "consistent" error.

Luria's findings are supported by investigations at the Haskins Laboratories in the United States. One of their reports (Liberman, et al., 1967) sums up their observations as follows:

The conclusion that there is a speech mode, and that it is characterized by processes different from those underlying the perception of other sounds, is strengthened by recent indications that speech and nonspeech sounds are processed primarily in different hemispheres of the brain.

Related Problems: Defective Storage (Memory)

Developmentally aphasic children can, fortunately, be trained to discriminate between isolated speech sounds (McReynolds, 1966) and to make correct discriminative responses when given an immediate opportunity to do so. However, his storage system may be defective for such signals. We often find that when even short periods of delay are introduced, many aphasic children seem unable to retain what they hear. In contrast to tasks for speech-sound discrimination, we usually find better performance for discrimination of other environmental sounds. The implication of these observations is that speech events call for different storage and control than do other auditory events. This, as we indicated above, is supported by the observations of the Haskins Laboratory investigators.

Defective Capacity for the Discrimination and Perception of Sounds in Contextual Utterance

A child may be able to discriminate and match isolated speech sounds, or even two or three phoneme units, especially if they contain a medial vowel (CVC), but still be unable to make the necessary discriminations and perceptions when sounds are incorporated into a normal utterance. We are aware that in a flow of speech, individual sounds are modified by their position in the utterance. Thus the *t* of *tin* is different from the *t* of *hits,* or of *bent,* or of *city.* The two *t*'s in *twenty* are perhaps as much different as they are alike, depending in part on whether the speaker is British or American, or is speaking "trippingly on the tongue" or in a lax and relaxed manner. Nevertheless, despite all of these differences, nonaphasic children somehow manage to recognise them all as /t/. Those of us who have studied phonetics will refer to each of the *t*'s as allophones of the phoneme /t/. Aphasic children seem to lack the ability to generalize the "members of a family of sounds" into phonemic categories. Instead, we speculate, they may try to store each sound as a discrete category-entity. The innumerable sounds a child must then store may not permit him to make matchings to a broad enough category to be of practical and functional use in speech processing. So an aphasic child may be impaired because he is a victim of too many, too narrow, too rigid, and possibly too precocious a hardening of phonemic categories. He may overload his storage system with too much phonetic junk and not end up with a basic set of categories. For American English, most of us get along with about 40 or so categories (phonemes).

DEVELOPMENTAL APHASIA: A DEFINITION

We shall be using the term *developmental aphasia* (congenital aphasia, dyslogia) to refer to the impairment for a child to acquire symbols for a language system. The impairment must be of sufficient degree to interfere with the child's ability to communicate. The use of the term developmental aphasia, or one of its synonyms, implies that the child's perceptual abilities for auditory (speech) events underlies his impairment for the acquisition of auditory symbols. His expressive disturbances are a manifestation of his intake or decoding impairment. A child cannot produce language if he cannot decode the speech to which he is exposed, or if the speech remains for him sounds without sense. An aphasic child may, in addition, have dysarthria and dyspraxia, impairments in the ability to control his articulatory mechanism, to make it do his bidding, for the amount of language he is able to take in— process and decode. These productive impairments are not, per se, aphasic but are motor difficulties which, unfortunately, may aggravate his problem for communication. We shall consider these impairments separately.

Minimal Brain Damage and Minimal Brain Dysfunction

On the basis of their behavior, positive and negative, and on the basis of their difficulties with learning, many developmentally aphasic children fall under the broad category of minimal brain dysfunction. We accept the position of Clements (1966, pp. 6–7) that "certain categories of deviant behavior, developmental dyscrasias, learning disabilities, and visual-motor-perceptual irregularities" are valid indices of brain dysfunctioning. "They represent neurological signs of a most meaningful kind, and reflect disorganized central nervous system functioning at the highest level." Thus, though it is frequently possible to demonstrate by the usual clinical neurological examination that perhaps 30 percent or more of developmentally aphasic children are clearly neurologically impaired, the majority of such children do not present such evidence. Most do, however, present behavioral indications, and especially language-learning difficulties, that do implicate the nervous system. So if we consider learning and behavior as expressions of central nervous system function, deviant behavior and learning disabilities in children who are not mentally retarded or severely impaired in their sensory mechanisms should, we believe, be considered indicative of central nervous system dysfunctioning. For such children we consider the term minimal brain dysfunction and the implication of minimal brain damage as quite appropriate.

The syndrome of minimal brain dysfunction refers to children who are not mentally retarded and who may, in fact, be near average or even above average in intellectual potential, but who present deviations in perceptual functioning, in conceptualization, in severe delay in language development, in attention, memory, and in control of attention. They may also show impulsivity and poor motor functioning. Since all these deviations are not necessarily present in all children, it is not a fixed and altogether stable syndrome. However, many if not most of the components of the syndrome are usually manifest in most of the children. The component of severe language retardation is, of course, necessary for our concept of the developmentally aphasic child.

Expressive Disturbances in Oral Apraxia

As we suggested earlier, we believe that virtually all expressive disturbances of developmentally aphasic children have their etiology in their intake impairment. Children must first understand before they can speak in the sense of using a language code. There are, however, some children—a very few—who despite evidence of their understanding of language nevertheless have severe impairment in expression. Such children, though sometimes designated as expressive aphasics, are much more likely to be ones with oral apraxia.

The child with oral apraxia usually does understand as much language as the parents claim. His developmental history is likely to reveal that he was normally responsive to environmental sounds as well as to human sounds. As an infant and young child, he was able to learn baby games, to clap hands on signal, and play peek-a-boo. Perhaps even before he was a year old, he could point to parts of the body when named by a parent and perform in various ways to verbal cues that provided the child and the parent with considerable pleasure. It is quite likely that until the child was 15 months old, the parents were not particularly concerned about his lack of speech. The parents quite properly began to show concern when the child, despite his increased comprehension of language, could not say any intelligible words. The parents might well have been advised by a pediatrician to be patient, that perhaps by 20 months, or surely by 24 months, the child's speech attempts would be intelligible. Perhaps by that time the child had achieved "ma-ma" or "da-da," but little more.

The early developmental history of the understanding-but-not-speaking child may reveal some of the following which we consider significant. As an infant, he may have cried somewhat more than his siblings at the same age. Early vocal play that ordinarily includes self-sound imitation (lalling) was absent. Echolalia, the imitation of sounds of an adult, was also absent. The parents may also recall that the child may have been a feeding problem as an infant. He seemed to prefer liquid and soft foods to any that required chewing. He may have regurgitated more often than his siblings, and he may have been regarded as a "lazy" chewer. This reputation is often maintained when the child is five or six years of age. All of these may be indications that the child had difficulty in establishing the synergy of oral movements required for mastication and swallowing, and suggest a congenital oral apraxia.

The developmental difficulties we have identified are not likely to be associated with difficulty in hearing or in auditory discrimination. What the child is unable to do is to monitor his oral mechanism, and particularly his organs of articulation, to do his bidding. An examination of the peripheral speech mechanism is likely to reveal that the child has difficulty in executing (imitating) movements with his articulators. Tongue pointing, lip licking, rapid tongue wagging may present difficulties, especially if repeated, fast movements are required. Such movements may be executed slowly, and often show improvement when the child's imitations can be performed before a mirror so that he can observe his own movements as well as those he is imitating. However, difficulties increase if the child is asked to repeat a sequence of movements such as "ip-ik-it" or "ba-da-ga."

By age three or four, the productive speech of these children is likely to be characterized by severe distortions of all or most non-visible sounds of speech. Lip sounds and single vowels are the most proficient combinations. Monosyllabic words that incorporate such sounds as "ma," "moo," and "be" may be intelligible. Even these may suffer, however, when an attempt is made to include them in a phrase or a sentence. In general, sequential sound making is severely impaired. Speech melody, however, is likely to be well established. This ability sometimes enables a child to communicate an idea if he can incorporate a key monosyllabic word or words in a phrase that, as a whole, is properly intoned. Although these children clearly have productive speech disturbance, we consider that the underlying disorder is an oral apraxia rather than an expressive aphasia. The child with oral apraxia cannot order his articulators to do his bidding. His understanding of language and the images of words are not impaired. The difficulty is motor and mechanical rather than a symbolic-linguistic impairment.

It is, of course, possible that a child may be both developmentally aphasic and orally apraxic. This compounds the child's difficulties, because even as he begins to improve in auditory discrimination and perception and understands spoken language, he cannot express his understanding through conventional speech or reinforce his perceptions with motor activities. He continues to be somewhat like the infant whose early understanding of speech is considerably beyond his ability to produce intelligible language. Unfortunately, when he is beyond the age of the infant, he as well as his parents will experience frustration because of his productive difficulties.

Expressive Impairments in Developmental Aphasia

As the developmentally aphasic child begins to acquire speech, his productions lag behind his understanding. In a sense he, too, is like the infant who understands many words before he can produce his own first words, and many sentence formulations before he utters a two- or three-word phrase-sentence, or one with recognizable syntax. He may still find some words elusive and may occasionally appear to be suffering from dysnomia. As he gains control over his word inventory, he must still develop his grammar (syntax). During this process, which most normal-speaking children have under fair control by age three, he may still seem to be hunting for words when he is really reaching for a formulation of words —a sentence. The child is quite likely to speak agrammatically, omitting functional words and grammatical markers before he utters his first "conventional" sentence. These are indeed expressive disturbances. As we indicated earlier in our description of the developmentally aphasic child in many ways his profile of language competencies appear to be a retarded shadow of his age peer. The shadow profile, however, is not smooth. It may reveal jagged irregularities which, in time, may smooth and eventually parallel that of his age peer, especially if there is no discrepancy between chronological and mental age.

REFERENCES

Brown, S. F., in Johnson, W., *et al.*, *Speech Handicapped School Children*, New York, Harper and Row, 1967.

Clements, S. D., "Minimal Brain, Dysfunction in Children," NINDB monograph, no. 3, U.S. Department of Health, Education, and Welfare, 1966.

Critchley, M., "Aphasiological Nomenclature and Definitions," *Cortex*, 3, 1, 1967, 3–25.

Eisenson, J., "Developmental Aphasia (Dyslogia): A Postulation of a Unitary Concept of the Disorder," *Cortex*, 4, 1968, 184–200.

———, "Developmental Aphasia: A Speculative View with Therapeutic Implications," *Journal of Speech and Hearing Disorders*, 33, 1, 1968, 3–13.

———, "Developmental Patterns of Non-Verbal Children," *Journal of Neurological Sciences*, 3, 1966a, 313–320.

———, "Perceptual Disturbances in Children with Central Nervous System Disfunctions and Implications for Language Development," *British Journal of Disorders of Communications*, 1, 1, 1966b, 21–32.

———, and Ogilvie, M., *Speech Correction in the Schools*, 3rd ed., 1971, chap. 16.

Forrest, T., Eisenson, J., and Stark, J., "EEG Findings in 113 Nonverbal Children," abstract in *Electroencephalographic Clinical Neurophysiology*, 22, 1967, 291.

Goldstein, R., Landau, W. M., and Kleffner, F. R., "Neurologic Assessment of Deaf and Aphasic Children," *Transactions of the American Otologic Society*, 46, 1958, 122–136.

Hardy, W. G., in Money, J., ed., *Reading Disability*, Baltimore, Johns Hopkins Press, 1962.

Kephart, N. C., *The Slow Learner in the Classroom*, New York, Merrill, 1960.

Lenneberg, E. H., *Biological Foundations of Language*, New York, Wiley, 52–72.

Liberman, A. M., Cooper, F. S., Shankweiler, D. P., and Studdert-Kennedy, M., "Perception of the Speech Code," *Psychological Review*, 74, 1967, 431–461.

Luria, A. R., *The Higher Cortical Functions of Man*, New York, Basic Books, 1966.

McReynolds, L. K., "Operant Conditioning for Investigating Speech Sound Discrimination in Aphasic Children," *Journal of Speech and Hearing Research*, 9, 1966, 519–528.

Morley, M. E., "Developmental and Receptive Expressive Aphasia," *Speech Pathology and Therapy*, 3, 64, 1960.

Assessment of Nonverbal [Severely Linguistically Retarded] Children

The primary purposes in the assessment of children who are severely delayed in their linguistic development are to determine the factors related to the delay and the implications of these factors, if they can be determined, for treatment. The information obtained from these evaluations has both immediate and future values. The immediate values should help make decisions on how to initiate a training and educational program for the child who is being assessed. The future values are related to the accumulation of a body of knowledge about children with severe language impairment which, hopefully, may permit better classification of categories, and so more heuristic educational "guesses" than are presently possible. In this

Chapter 5

chapter we shall address ourselves primarily to the first of these objectives.

In all assessment procedures it is essential that the clinician observe and note how *the results of the evaluation are obtained as well as* what *is obtained.* All results should be considered tentative, thus implying that evaluations must be repeated periodically and that impressions should not be fixed after an initial trial, however productive it may seem to be, of an evaluation. Moreover, all assessments should include a period of training to permit the clinical team to learn whether and how, at a given time and under a given set of conditions, the child shows what he is capable of learning.

Pediatric-Neurological Assessment

In broad terms, the pediatric-neurological assessment should provide us with information about how the child is functioning as a physical being and with information for making decisions and recommendations as to what other medical examinations may be required to complete the work-up.

The specialized contribution of the pediatric neurologist is, of course, concerned with determining the integrity or impairments of the child's neurosensory system. Clement's "Minimal Brain Dysfunction in Children" (1966) provides a guideline for the medical evaluation of deviating children and details the responsibilities of the physician in the diagnostic assessment of deviating children. The guidelines include the following:

1. Medical history:
   a. "To include pre-, peri-, and post-natal information. Details of all childhood illnesses should be obtained, including age of child at time of illness, symptoms, severity, course and care (such as physician in attendance, hospitalization)."
   b. Developmental—"To include details of motor, language, adaptive, and personal–social development."
   c. Family–Social—"To involve parents, child, and others as indicated. The family–social history should include detailed information regarding family constellation, acculturation factors, specific inter-personal family dynamics, emotional stresses, and traumata."

2. Physical examination:
   a. General—"To evaluate general physical status and to search for systemic disease. The physical examination should be done as part of the current evaluation of the child. . . ."[1]
   b. Neurologic—"To evaluate neurological function and to search for specific disorders of the nervous system. The developmental aspects of neurological integration assume primary importance for this examination, especially with reference to integrated motor acts as opposed to simple reflexes."[2]

Special additional examinations for the deviant child include ophthalmologic, otologic, psychiatric, and whatever other evaluations the pediatrician considers necessary, based upon the information and impressions he obtains during his evaluation. In addition, the pediatrician may request laboratory work-up for blood and urine analysis.

The pediatric neurologist routinely assesses the child's motor status by observations of walking, standing, the child's awareness of body sense and his "relationship of himself in space," the child's sense of balance (eyes open and closed), and his expression of laterality (hand, foot, eye).

It is obvious that a medical assessment such as outlined above cannot be completed in the usual comparatively short period of a routine office visit to a physician. At the Stanford University Institute for Childhood Aphasia, the pediatrician spends at least two half days, and whatever additional time may be necessary, for his pediatric-neurologic assessment. Whenever possible he also accompanies the child for the electroencephalographic evaluation.

Part of the responsibilities of the pediatrician is to interpret the results of the examination to the parents, insofar as such information will help in the understanding and treatment of the child. Similarly, the medical data are reported to the other mem-

---

[1]At the Institute for Childhood Aphasia, Stanford University School of Medicine, we follow the practice, which we believe to be common, of obtaining the results of past examinations from the child's (family) physician and conducting our own examination for the child's current status.

[2]The Institute for Childhood Aphasia routinely includes an EEG evaluation.

bers of the assessment team and, of course, included in the written summaries in each child's case history.

PSYCHOLOGICAL ASSESSMENT

Much of the assessment of the clinical psychologist is, in effect, an extension of the work of the pediatrician and so may be considered as part of an extended neurological or, perhaps better, a neuropsychological evaluation. The guidelines shown in Clement's article include the following as the core of the psychological evaluation:

1. "Individual comprehensive assessment of intellectual functioning."
2. "Measures of complex visual-motor-perceptual functioning."
3. "Behavioral observations in a variety of settings."
4. "Additional indices of learning and behavior as indicated."

In regard to the first guideline, it is probably better to consider the assessment of intellectual functioning as one to estimate potential or capacity to learn. Presumably, a nonverbal child's potential is greater than his immediate manifest ability. Emphasis, we believe, should be on tests and procedures which do not require verbal mediation. Fortunately, there are many standardized tests that may be administered without oral language, and others that may be adapted for use with nonverbal and severely language-delayed children. Among the tests we have found useful at the Institute for Childhood Aphasia are the following.

Gesell Developmental Schedule (Gessell, 1949) ;[3]

Cattell Infant Intelligence Scale (Cattell, 1947) .[4]

The above two inventories estimate intellectual potential based on the motor and perceptual development of the child.

[3]Full data for the cited tests will be found in the References at the end of this chapter. In a strict sense, the Gesell inventory is not a test of intelligence because it does not, as Darley (1964, p. 107) observes, directly sample behavior.

[4]The same observation holds for the Cattell scale. Anastasi (1958, p. 283) notes that "these schedules may be regarded as a refinement and elaboration of the qualitative observations routinely made by pediatricians."

The Bayley Scales of Infant Development (Bayley, 1969).

This index provides a considerable advance over the Gesell schedules. The Bayley scales are intended for the assessment of early mental and psychomotor development of babies and young children up to 30 months of age. These scales provide for differences based on age, sex, color, and urban–rural upbringing.

Scale Inventories

The Leiter International Performance Scale (Leiter, 1948);

The Columbia Mental Maturity Scale (Burgmeister et al., 1953).

The above two inventories—by gesture, pantomime, and demonstration—can be administered without the use of oral language. The early items of these inventories call for perceptual discrimination and/or matchings and do not require abstraction or conceptualization. They are, therefore, particularly applicable for children below age four or five who are severely impaired in language development.

The Raven Progressive Matrices (Raven, 1962);

Porteus Maze Test (Porteus, 1965).

Both of these inventories call for the subject to solve perceptual problems through simple motor acts. The tasks in the Raven matrices require the subject to solve problems which are presented in abstract designs and figures. They become quite complicated at the upper levels. The Porteus maze inventory requires the subject to find his way out of a maze diagram, using a pencil and the maze diagrams to show the solution.

Ammons Full-Range Picture Vocabulary Test (Ammons and Ammons, 1958);

Peabody Picture Vocabulary Test, Forms A and B (Dunn, 1965).

The Ammons and the Peabody inventories assess intelligence through the use of pictures on cards and key words presented by the examiner. The basic task for the child is to point to the picture that goes with the presented (spoken) key word. No verbal response is required but, of course, the child must have some understanding of language for the test to be relevant. These scales will be considered later in our discussion of language assessment.

Form Board Tests

There are a number of adaptations and variations of form board tests based, for the most part, on the original Seguin form boards. The Arthur Point Scale (1947) includes adaptations of Seguin form boards as part of a scale of performance tests. These may be easily employed with children with severe language impairment. The Gesell Form Board (1940) is a revision of an earlier model developed at the Vineland Training School. The Gesell Form Board (1952) is especially appropriate for younger children or for ones suspected of being mentally retarded. It requires the insertation of three forms—a circle, a triangle, and a square—each approximately three inches in diameter, into an opening in a board.

Visual Perceptual Tests

Visual perceptual and perceptual-motor tests have a long history. Their development and employment are related to the need to find tasks that can be administered to individuals who have a limited understanding of language or an impairment for the reception of oral language. Practically, also, visual tasks (the perception of visual events) can be administered because, unlike auditory events, they are stable rather than ephemeral. The nature of the performance required can be demonstrated, and the administration—the directions—can be given in pantomime. Several visual-perceptual tests are included in scaled tests of intelligence, such as the Wechsler batteries, the Stanford-Binet (Terman and Merrill, 1960), and the Merrill–Palmer (Stutsman, 1931). We shall confine our discussion to tests in frequent use.

The Bender Visual-Motor Gestalt Test (Bender, 1938).

This test requires drawings by the subject to assess visual perception. The stimulus items are nine line-drawing figures presented one at a time to the subject for copying. Bender found that brain-damaged subjects perform in characteristically different ways (produce different kinds of figures and make different kinds of errors) from normal and emotionally disturbed subjects. Norms for assessment of the drawings of young children have been developed by Koppitz (1964). It is, of course, essential that the clinician take into account any motor disability a child may have in his execution of the drawings. We have found that some children who are unable to copy (reproduce) a satisfactory drawing may nevertheless show their perceptual competence in a match-to-sample (multiple-choice) situation. So, it is possible in clinical assessment to separate the visual-perceptual aspect of the task from the motor aspect, and therefore to avoid an assumption that a distorted or different product necessarily represents the child's perception of the stimulus event.

Block-Design Tests.

Wechsler, among others, includes block-design tasks as part of his performance scales. The original Kohs block designs (1923) included figures (designs) made up with the colors red, yellow, blue, and white. Modifications such as Wechsler's reduce the colors to red and white, and to relatively simple designs.

Block-design tasks require that the subject be able to perceive a pattern or design of different colors as a *gestalt*, or whole configuration; to analyze the pattern into component parts; and to reproduce the pattern, presented on a card, by an arrangement of colored blocks.

The standard method for administering the block-design tests is to present a card with the design—the stimulus item—and several colored blocks. The patient is expected to arrange the blocks so that the result (the top colors on the blocks) reproduce the design. The procedure should be illustrated once, or more, for the subject. If the subject fails, we recommend that a block arrangement rather than a card be used for reproduction—copying. If this is done successfully, then the card design should be tried again, with a second demonstration.

In testing young children we recommend that only simple designs be used and that the colors be limited to two, as in the Wechsler Intelligence Scale for Children (1949) and the Wechsler Pre-School and Primary Scale of Intelligence (1967).

Other tests of visual perception, which are included in many general inventories of intelligence, include the ability to draw a cross, a square, or a diamond.

Frostig Developmental Test of Visual Perception (Frostig et al., 1964).

The Frostig is designed to assess five operationally defined visual-perceptual functions: visual-motor coordination, figure-ground perception, perceptual constancy (the perception of invariant properties such as shape, size, and position despite the variability of sensory impressions), position in space, and spatial relationships.

By this inventory, according to the authors, a clinician can chart a child's strengths and weaknesses in visual perception and therewith constitute the basis of a remedial program.

As a diagnostic instrument, the Frostig test is helpful in directing attention to possible visual-perceptual impairments or delays in children of primary-school age. However, the clinician must be certain that the child understands the task necessary for an appropriate performance.

Knox Cube Imitation Test (Grace Arthur Modification).

This test is included in the Arthur Point Scale of Performance Tests, Revised Form II (1947).

The Knox cube test calls for the imitation of a sequence of block tapping movements on four blocks. The test begins with a sequence of two taps (1–4) and progresses finally to a sequence of seven taps (4–1–3–4–2–1–4). The test can be administered with verbal directions, "Now you do what I did," or by imitation without verbal direction. It constitutes a basis for assessing visual sequencing through a simple motor response.

Motor Assessment

In the assessment of the child with serious language delay it is essential that we learn how the child is functioning motorically at the time of our evaluation. Specifically, we need to know whether the child has the motor capabilities for speech production. Such assessment may, in part, be done by direct observation of the child's peripheral speech mechanism—the size and shape of his oral cavity and his articulatory organs, the arrangement of his jaws and teeth, and the ability of the child to produce isolated and sequential movements of his articulation at a rate approximating what is needed in speech. Observations of this sort are made by the pediatric neurologist and by the language (speech) clinician.

Important additional information is provided by observations of the child's gross and fine body movements. The child's manner of walking, hopping, skipping, jumping, etc., his ability to balance on one foot, and his ability to throw and catch a ball or bean bag, or even to bounce a ball, provide us with information about eye–hand coordination as well as of his spatial orientation. Laterality development, which should include eye, foot, and ear preference, as well as hand preference, are now items of increased importance for language clinicians because of the correlations between the establishment of laterality preference, cerebral dominance, and language development. Information on present laterality preference may be obtained as part of the medical examination or as additional assessments by one of the other members of the evaluation team. Guided observations may be made through the use of specially devised tests such as the Oseretsky Test of Motor Proficiency (Doll, 1947) and the Harris Tests of Lateral Dominance (1955).

The Oseretsky test is a scale of six separate tests with separate items according to the subject's age. The scale measures general static coordination, dynamic coordination of the hands, general dynamic coordination, motor speech, simultaneous voluntary movements, and asynkinesia (ability to perform without overflow or superfluous movements).

The Harris test is, despite its name, an inventory to assess expressions of developed lateral preference. It includes a number of items requiring simultaneous and coordinated movements of both hands. The principle on which the Harris test is based is that when both hands attempt to perform the same movement simultaneously, the nonpreferred hand (Harris uses the term "the non dominant hand") tends to execute a mirrorwise or reverse action of the preferred hand. Hand preference, and so presumably cerebral dominance, is measured by the number of reversals or partial reversals made by either hand. Preference (dominance) is assessed on the basis of the number of reversals for the various acts involved. Young children, those below age four or five, are not expected to be able to perform on all items of the Harris test.

Social Development

The child's social development is another aspect of the psychological assessment. For most children language acquisition and social maturity are intimately related. For children with severe language impairment this relationship does not hold. Parents are the primary assessors of the child's social and emotional development. The Vineland and the Pre-School Attainment Record are basically questionnaire inventories which provide the interviewer with information to form judgments about the child's social development.

The Vineland Social Maturity Scale (Doll, 1965).

This scale was designed to assess successive stages of social competence from infancy to adult life. In essence, it is a series of items arranged in age periods (levels). The informant provides the interviewer with information relative to aspects of motor and perceptual development in the early years and to social competence during adolescence and adult life. When applied to children, it affords a basis for developmental assessment. Items such as the child's ability to laugh, imitate sounds (first level), name familiar objects (second level), and toilet habits (second and third levels) help the examiner to arrive at clinical judgments about the child. The nature of the scale, which requires parental recall of the child's performances, lends itself to error. Parental reports may be compared with actual performances of the present status of the child to provide some insight about parental judgments. Although the scale is intended to yield a social quotient, the clinical implications about the specifics of what the child is or is not doing according to age expectancy are probably of greater importance.

The Preschool Attainment Record (PAR) (Doll, 1966).

This is intended as a supplement and extension of the Vineland Social Maturity Scale. Although the PAR has not been normatively standardized, the scale does permit comparisons of siblings within a family, or comparisons of the child with himself over periods of time. The PAR covers a range of half-year intervals from birth to seven years for eight aspects of physical, social, and intellectual development—ambulation, manipulation, rapport, communication, responsibility, information, ideation, and creativity. The appraisal is conducted by interview with a parent or other informant with dependable knowledge about the child's developmental history. The information thus obtained may be supplemented by direct observation of the child if he is available and accessible. A record form is provided for a summary and profile.

Behavioral Characteristics

Among behavioral signs and characteristics that are frequently associated with brain damage and which, therefore, may be prognostic of aphasia in the child with severe language delay are the following: hyperactivity, especially as an accompaniment of failure in performance; perceptual-motor impairments; poor perceptual integration, especially for multiple-sensory stimuli; disorders of attention (short attention span and "morbidity" of attention expressed in perseverative responses and disinclination to disengage from a present task); poor memory span, especially for auditory events; emotional lability; impulsivity; and distractibility.

Audiological Assessment

The routine audiometric evaluation is only a small part of what we need to learn from the audiologist in regard to the hearing *and* listening capacities of the aphasic child. Many aphasic children are known to have some degree of hearing loss as determined by routine pure-tone audiometry. Unless such hearing loss is moderately severe or severe (above 60 dB in the "crucial" pitch range), a report that is limited to results of pure-tone signal assessment is of little value. What we need to know is the child's reception for speech and his ability to perceive and to discriminate speech signals, vowels, consonants, and combinations of vowels and consonants. We also need to know whether the child responds to a signal when it is presented initially, and then "adapts" and ceases to respond on the second or third presentation of the same signal. Further, we need to know whether there is any evidence of perceptual "deafness" to some signals and not to others. If, for example, the audiologist obtains a reliable threshold of response for a pure-tone signal, but an inconsistent response to speech signals, we are then provided with information which tells us something about the child's capacity for listening as well as for hearing.

Additional assessment is needed of the child's ability to sequence a series of speech signals, e.g., not only to determine the child's auditory memory span for consonant–vowel (CV) combinations but also his ability to keep the order of the phonemic presentations in mind so that he can discriminate between consonant–vowel (CV) versus a second combination of consonant–vowel or vowel–consonant. The number of phonemes a child can process correctly, through either a matching or oral reproduction (if the child is capable of the latter), helps to shed light on what the auditory perceptual abilities of the child are and provides a basis for where training needs to begin.

The audiologist cannot expect to assess a child suspected of being aphasic as quickly as he can most other children. The audiologist must anticipate the need for some conditioning training as well as for teaching the child how to respond to the presented auditory stimuli. The audiologist must be patient, resourceful, seductive, and yet firm in getting his child–patient involved in the task of assessment. As with all other members of the evaluation team, the audiologist needs to report not only the results obtained but also the conditions under which they were obtained. His clinical observations and judgments are as important as his objective findings.

To sum up, the audiological evaluation for a child with severe language delay who may be aphasic must provide information about his sensory reception to auditory signals and, probably more important, about his perception (phonemic discrimination and sequencing) for the special kind of auditory events that constitute speech.

LANGUAGE ASSESSMENT

The language clinician has a key and overlapping role with the psychologist and audiologist in the assessment of a child with severe language delay. In the broadest terms, the language clinician is expected to determine, by formal examinations and by observation, at what levels the child is able to function relative to his comprehension and production of language. More specifically, the language clinician assesses the child's competences and performance in regard to his phonemic proficiencies (the sounds and sound combinations he can discriminate and process), his morphemic proficiencies (the way he combines sounds into words), his lexical proficiencies (words he knows and those he can produce according to "sample" conditions), and the child's syntactic proficiency (the level of sentence he can understand and produce in his own utterances).

At the present time, the language clinician has fewer standardized test instruments available to him than does the psychologist for his assessments. There are, fortunately, a few standardized instruments which may be used by the language clinician in his evaluation.

Auditory Discrimination and Perception

Normal language acquisition requires the ability to process signals that are received by our distance receptors—our eyes and our ears. The special character of speech signals and the knowledge we now have about the processing of such signals by the central nervous system are still meager and limited. Thus, we cannot as yet expect to have reliable tools and measurements for the assessment of perceptual functions that underlie speech perception. Tests such as digit span, which is included in most inventories or scales for the assessment of intelligence, are of no use in the evaluation of a truly nonverbal child. Children with some language ability may be assessed with such items as digit span, nonsense syllable span, and with the widely used Wepman test.

The Wepman Auditory Discrimination Test (Wepman, 1958).

This test consists of 40 single-syllable word pairs, 10 of which are identical, e.g., ball-ball, and 30 of which differ by a single phoneme, e.g., bum-bun. The subject is asked to indicate whether the pairs are the same or different. The score is based on the number of errors made.

The Boston University Speech Sound Discrimination Picture Test (Pronovost and Dumbleton, 1955).

This test employs word pairs differing by one phoneme, e.g., dish-fish, and pictures to assess speech-sound discrimination. Three sets of pictures are presented on each test page. The child is directed to point to the picture pairings that represent the word pairs. The score for speech-sound discrimination is based on the total number of correct identifications. The authors of the test consider a child to have average or normal speech-sound discrimination if he makes 65 correct responses out of a total of 72. A score below 59 indicates poor ability for speech-sound discrimination.

Other tests for speech-sound discrimination which may be used with children with some language ability include phonetically balanced (PB) word lists and spondee words (two-syllable words with equal stress on each syllable). These tests are usually administered by an audiologist and constitute part of routine speech hearing examination. The tests are not, however, usually applicable to preschool children or to children with severe language retardation.

Receptive-Language Ability

The Peabody Picture Vocabulary Test (Dunn, 1965) and the Ammons Full-Range Picture Vocabulary Test (Ammons and Ammons, 1958), which were discussed briefly earlier, provide a basis for determining a child's receptive-language vocabulary through the use of standardized instruments. As indicated earlier, a nonverbal response—pointing—is all that is required of the examinee. The nature of these scales is such that it can readily be administered by a language clinician who has had no specific training in psychological test administration. The language clinician learns from the results of either the Peabody (PPVT) or the Ammons how a child, on the basis of a sampling of vocabulary, compares with other children of his age. Thus, a receptive-language age or, more properly, a receptive-vocabulary age or level can be approximated.

The Picture Speech Discrimination Test (Mecham and Jex, 1962).

This test employs words selected from the Thorndike–Lorge list of high-frequency terms in a picture–word matching task. The test includes 86 cards, each having three pictures. One of the pictures is a correct match for the card. The other two words are acoustically similar to the names of the other pictures. The child is instructed to point to the correct picture, that is, the picture which is correct for *one* of the three words spoken by the examiner.

Articulation (Phonemic Proficiency)

Between ages seven and eight most children have control of the sounds of their language system. Table 3, which is based on

Templin's data (1957) is a summary of the phonemic development of children between the ages of three and seven.

TABLE 3. Age at Which 75 Percent of Children First Uttered Various Types of Sounds Correctly

Chronological Age	Sounds
3	Initial, medial, and final nasals; initial, medial plosives; initial, medial semivowels; vowels; diphthongs
4	Final plosives
5	Final semivowels; final combinations; initial double-consonant blends*
6	Initial, medial, final fricatives; final double-consonant blends; reversed triple-consonant blends; reversed double-consonant blends
7	Initial, final, triple-consonant blends

Source: Templin (1957).

*Examples of blend: *pl* forms an initial consonant blend sound in *play; bl* is a consonant blend in *blue; st* is a sound blend in *stop; cl* is a consonant blend in *clean.*

The list that follows gives the average age for the control of 24 consonants of English (Templin, 1957, p. 53).

Sound	Age	Sound	Age
m	3	r	4
n	3	s	4.5
ng	3	sh	4.5
p	3	ch	4.5
f	3	t	6
h	3	th	6
w	3	v	6
y	3.5	l	6
k	4	th (voiced)	7
b	4	z	7
d	4	zh	7
g	4	j	7

There are numerous published tests for the assessment of a child's articulatory proficiency. Among the most widely used are the standardized tests by Templin and Darley (1960). The long form of the test contains 176 items. Pictures are used to elicit responses (naming of the picture for the key sound as well as for sound blends). The child may also complete a sentence calling for the use of the key word or repeat the word (elicited imitation) spoken by the examiner. An evaluation is also made of the child's articulatory proficiency (intelligibility) in conversational speech. Templin and Darley provide norms for children by age and sex, so that the individual child tested may be compared with the standardized scores based on the number of sounds correctly produced.

The short form of the Templin–Darley tests comprises 50 items and is intended as a screening device. If a child makes errors for a particular sound, then the test items from the longer test should be used.

McDonald (1964) is the author of *A Deep Test of Articulation.* McDonald's test is based on the principle that a syllable rather than a discrete sound is the basic unit in articulatory coding. Pictures are used in pairs to "connect" syllables so that combinations such as *tubvase, tubsheep* and *teethsheep* may be elicited. Each sound is tested in combinations which McDonald considers to be *fundamental phonetic contexts*. A score sheet and instructions are provided to determine the child's percentage of correct articulation. The McDonald approach, because it does "deep test," is useful as a diagnostic instrument for articulatory proficiency in brief contextual utterance. The nature of the procedure requires more training of the subject than does the Templin–Darley or most other published tests.

Templin constructed a speech-sound discrimination test for use in her study of the development of language skills in children. The test, designed especially for preschool age children "is based on the identification of similarity and difference in the acoustic value of familiar words which can be pictured" (1957, p. 14). The stimulus situations are cards with pairs of pictures of familiar objects whose common names are words which are similar in pronunciation except for single-sound elements; e.g., *clocks* and *blocks, bell* and *ball.* The child is directed to point to the picture denoted by the word presented by the examiner. Fifty-nine pictured word pairs are employed in the test. The list of words and directions for administration and scoring are described by Templin (1957, pp. 14, 63ff, and 159).

Scaled Inventories for Receptive and Productive Language

The Illinois Test of Psycholinguistic Abilities (ITPA), revised edition (Kirk, McCarthy, and Kirk, 1968).

"The psycholinguistic model on which the ITPA is based attempts to relate those functions whereby the intentions of an individual are transmitted (verbally or nonverbally) to another individual and, reciprocally, functions whereby the environment or the intentions of another individual are received and interpreted" *(ITPA, Examiner's Manual,* p. 7). The model of the ITPA postulates three dimensions of cognitive abilities:

1. *Channels of communication*—these are the routes or sensory modalities "through which the content of communication flows." The ITPA deals specifically with the auditory and visual input modalities; the tests of the ITPA assess for expression of input through the auditory-vocal, auditory-motor, visual-motor, and visual-vocal approaches.

2. *Psycholinguistic processes*—Three main processes are considered in analyzing the child's language acquisition. These are (1) *the receptive process,* or the ability of the child to recognize and understand what has been presented to him orally; (2) the expressive process, or the skills requisite to the expression of ideas by either vocal (oral) or visible (gesture) performance; and (3) the "organizing process which involves the internal manipulation of percepts, concepts, and linguistic symbols. It is a central mediating process elicited by the receptive process and preceding the expressive process."

3. *Levels of organization*—These are determined by the degree "to which habits of communication are organized within the individual. . . ." The ITPA model postulates two levels: (1) the representational, which calls upon the established complex mediating process of utilizing symbols (verbal mediation) that "carry the meaning of an object," and (2) the automatic level, which calls

upon less voluntary but highly automatic functions. Such automatic functions or expressions of a "chain of responses" are involved in activities such as visual and auditory closure, speed of perception, ability to reproduce a sequence presented visually or orally, rote learning, the synthesizing of isolated sounds into words, and utilizing (applying) the redundancies of experience. In essence, whether the test item is visual or auditory, the child is required on the basis of presumed exposure and experience to identify an event, e.g., an object partially concealed, or complete a verbal expression. Auditory-sequential memory is tested by digit span, with digits presented at one-half-second intervals. Visual sequencing is tested by requiring the child to reproduce an arrangement of nonmeaningful figures (chips) after a five-second exposure.

The ITPA is a standardized instrument which provides norms for children in the age ranges two years six months to ten years. A psycholinguistic age may be derived for each of the 12 subtests as well as for the test as a whole. A profile sheet is provided for entering the various scores, which permits the clinicians to make comparisons of the individual psycholinguistic abilities of the child.

The Northwestern Syntax Screening Test (NSST) (Lee, 1969 and 1970).

This test is intended, as the name implies, as a quick screening instrument to identify children "who are sufficiently delayed in syntactic development to warrant further study." The NSST assesses both receptive and productive (expressive) use of syntactic forms, using identical linguistic structures in both parts of the test.

Receptive items are tested by having the child point to pictures that correspond to a presented statement, e.g., "Show me *the cat is under the chair.*" "Now show me *the cat is behind the chair.*"

Expressive items are tested by adding the task of expression to the initial task of reception. The instructions call for the examiner to present the pictures by saying something along this line, "I will tell you about these pictures. When I am done, you copy me. Say just what I say. Don't talk until I tell you. Ready?" The examiner then shows the first page of pictures and says, *"The baby is sleeping. The baby is not sleeping.* Now, what's this picture?" The examiner points to the key picture *the baby is sleeping* and waits for the child to reply; then the examiner points to the other picture and waits for a reply.

The task for the expressive items is essentially that of *elicited imitation* with pictures used as a visual reinforcement. The scores are based on correct verbatim imitation of sentences or on responses which, though not verbatim reproductions, "accomplish the grammatical test item but which alter the sentence insignificantly and preserve grammatical correctness. . . ." The examiner should note all errors of omission or modification of the presented sentence.

Percentile ratings for receptive and expressive items are provided based on a population of 242 children ranging in age between three years and seven to eleven years. The children came from middle- and upper-class communities and from homes where a standard American dialect was spoken. According to the manual for the NSST, "Any child whose score is below the 10th percentile would warrant further study and a consideration for a remedial language training program, unless his performance in other language areas were satisfactory." The test author emphasizes that "it is important that the examiner consider this test a screening instrument only and not a detailed analysis of a child's syntactic skill."

Both the ITPA and the NSST are intended for children who have enough verbal behavior so that their productions can be evaluated. Neither of these instruments is applicable to preschool children with severe language retardation. The ITPA has been in wide use. The revised edition is accepted as a standardized test, which permits the clinician to make comparisons and judgment based on scale scores and standard scores with established norms. Thus, through the use of the ITPA when applicable—for children who though linguistically retarded can decode and encode language —it is possible to obtain a language age and specific language function scores.

The NSST is, in our view, an early and experimental approach to a new kind of language-assessment procedure. It is limited to assessment of syntax. With a larger and broader population sampling, which should result in revised norms and percentile scores, the value of the NSST should increase. At the present time it does have merit in providing a clinician with material for arriving at a guided judgment about a child's comprehension and performance relative to a number of syntactic formulations that differ in level and complexity.

Elicited Imitation

In our discussion of the NSST we indicated that the task for the expressive items was to elicit a syntactical construction from the child based on a verbal formulation. The pictures are employed as a visual reinforcement so that the child could be assumed to comprehend what he hears. Since the early 1960s the technique of elicited imitation (requesting the child to repeat verbal constructions) has been used as a shortcut approach to assess the child's syntactical production. The long approach, of course, is to take a number of samples of a child's spontaneous speech in a variety of settings so that the total inventory or corpus would be acceptable as representative of the child's syntactic proficiency. Findings such as those of Brown and Fraser (1963) indicated that in the range of 25 to 35 months, children's repetition (imitation) of presented adult sentences were found to have the same mean number of words and to have the same syntactic character as their spontaneous utterances stimulated the use of elicited imitation in the study of children's language. Somewhat older children, however (those between ages 37 and 43 months), were found by Fraser, Bellugi, and Brown (1963) to be able to imitate sentences which they could not comprehend. In using elicited imitation for the assessment of syntax in children under three years of age, and for children with severe language delay, we need not to be concerned with the matter of production without comprehension. Our assumption is that such children do, in fact, reveal their proficiency for syntax in their elicited imitative productions.

The key problem in the use of elicited imitation is to produce a series of model sentences that incorporate syntactical features according to a developmental schedule based on the syntactic development of normal children. The sentences used in the NSST represent one such effort. Another list in the published literature is that of Menyuk (1963). The use of sentences such as Lee's in the NSST and Menyuk's may provide information as to what syntactical construction a child is or is not able to manage. At the present time, however, such sentences and the elicited-imitation techniques do not provide us with established norms for syntactical proficiency.

Auditory Comprehension of Language Structure

An instrument to assess oral (auditory) language comprehension of language structure still in the experimental stage is described by Carrow (1968). The Carrow test consists of a set of cards, each of which contains one or more black-and-white line drawings. The pictures are designed to "represent referential categories and contrasts that can be signaled by form classes and function words, morphological constructions, grammatical categories, and syntactic structure." The child indicates his response by pointing to a line drawing on the stimulus card.

The Carrow test at present comprises 123 items. In scoring, each item is assigned a point value of one. The total score is the number of items passed (correct pointings). Tentative norms are provided at six-month intervals for children in the age range three to seven years.

Another experimental instrument to assess a child's language comprehension is the *Assessment of Children's Language Comprehension (ACLC)*, Research Edition (Foster, Giddan, and Stark, 1970). This test uses a core vocabulary of 50 common words which are combined into phrases of two, three, and four elements. Visual displays are employed for the child to identify (point to) the picture which is appropriate to the test phrase utterance spoken by the examiner. The ACLC attempts to assess (a) the child's receptive vocabulary for common words, (b) the number of critical elements (information words) he can process, and (c) the pattern in the breakdown (failures) of critical sequences.

The ACLC has three "critical" levels. On the first level, comprising picturable one- and two-syllable items, the child is required to identify common count nouns, the present progressive form of verbs, and some prepositions and adjectives. The second level introduces two critical items. A correct response is intended to reveal the child's understanding of the relationship of the items, e.g., "cat-walking" in a display that includes a cat walking, a cat sitting, a man sitting, and a horse walking. The third level includes three critical items with the addition of a preposition, e.g., "ball under the table."

The authors have found that the test can be administered in 10 to 15 minutes.

The ACLC is not a standardized scale and does not provide norms based on an age-distribution sampling of normal children. It is a clinical instrument, which provides information as to the specifics of the critical levels and elements described above. This information can be used as a basis for language training and for making individual comparisons as to the results of training. The preliminary forms of the ACLC have been used for these purposes at the Stanford Institute for Childhood Aphasia.

Trial Teaching

Perhaps the best assessment procedure and the testing of assessment is trial teaching. Optimally, if not practically, every child who is of the age and who does not have clear indications of sensory and motor disabilities which might explain failure for speech onset should be given several weeks of trial teaching. Routine testing, even if it is testing in depth and over a period of a week or more, assesses the results of the child's exposure, experiences, and influences up to the time of the formal assessment. Trial teaching adds a dimension of new experiences in a new setting with a different person. Under this new set of conditions the child himself may be helped to express his potentials rather than his limitations. Thus, a greater sampling of behavior may be assessed, and insights gained which may be of therapeutic significance in going beyond the findings of formal assessment. In the final analysis, the purposes of assessment for a child with severe language delay is to determine not only what he has acquired or has failed to acquire in language but also whether, what, and how he can acquire more with the intervention of "direct" instruction. This is the purpose of trial teaching.

Summary

We have described the roles and functions of professional personnel in the assessment of children who are severely retarded in language development, using as models the personnel who constitute the professional staff of the Institute for Childhood Aphasia at the Stanford University School of Medicine. We should like to emphasize, however, that except for the special contributions of the medical members, the roles and functions are not necessarily restricted along the lines described above. Roles may overlap and/or be shared. The only requirement in assessment that we feel needs to be strictly observed is that no person assumes a responsibility or function for which he has not been trained.

We have described a number of tests, scales, and approaches in assessment which, for the most part, we have had experience with and found useful. We are, of course, aware that other instruments and other approaches may be equally useful. Bangs (1968, chap. 4) describes her philosophy and the assessment tools for preschool age children with language and learning disorders. Another approach, intended primarily for children with multiple motor-perceptual problems and language disabilities, is described by Wyatt (1969, chap. 13). Berry (1969, chaps. 7 and 8) describes approaches and testing instruments and procedures for children with a wide range of language disabilities, but not for those whose impairments are so severe as to justify a designation of aphasia.

REFERENCES

Ammons, R. B., and Ammons, H. S., *The Full-Range Picture Vocabulary Test*, Missoula, Montana, Psychological Test Specialists, 1958.

Anastasi, A., *Differential Psychology*, 3rd ed., New York, Macmillan, 1958.

Arthur, G., *A Point Scale of Performance Tests*, Revised Form II, New York, Psychological Corporation, 1947.

Bangs, T. E., *Language and Learning Disorders of the Pre-Academic Child*, New York, Appleton-Century-Crofts, 1968.

Bayley, N., *The Bayley Scales of Infant Development*, New York, Psychological Corporation, 1969.

Bender, L., "A Visual–Motor Gestalt Test and Its Clinical Use," New York, American Orthopsychiatry Research Monograph no. 3, 1938.

Berry, M. F., *Language Disorders of Children*, New York, Appleton-Century-Crofts, 1969.

Brown, R., and Fraser, C., "The Acquisition of Syntax," in Cofer, C. N., and Musgrave, B. S., eds., *Verbal Behavior and Learning Problems and Processes*, New York, McGraw Hill, 1963, 158–197.

Burgmeister, B., Blum, L., and Lorge, I., *Columbia Mental Maturity Scale*, New York, Harcourt, Brace, and World, 1953.

Carrow, M. A., "The Development of Auditory Comprehension of Language Structure in Children," *Journal of Speech and Hearing Disorders*, 33, 1968, 99–111.

Cattell,, P., *The Measurement of Intelligence of Infants and Young Children,* New York, Psychological Corporation, 1947.

Clements, S. D., "Minimal Brain Dysfunction in Children," NINDB Monograph no. 3, U. S. Department of Health, Education, and Welfare, 1966.

Darley, F. L., *Diagnosis and Appraisal of Communication Disorders,* Englewood Cliffs, New Jersey, Prentice-Hall, 1964.

Doll, E. A., *Vineland Social Maturity Scale,* Circle Pines, Minnesota, American Guidance Service, 1965.

————, *Preschool Attainment Record,* Circle Pines, Minnesota, American Guidance Service, 1966.

————, ed., *The Oseretsky Test of Motor Proficiency,* Minneapolis, Educational Publishers, 1947.

Dunn, L. M., *Peabody Picture Vocabulary Test,* Nashville, American Guidance Service, 1965.

Foster, C. R., Giddan, J. J., and Stark, J., *Assessment of Children's Language Comprehension,* Palo Alto, California, Consulting Psychologists Press, 1970.

Fraser, D., Bellugi, U., and Brown, R., "Control of Grammar in Imitation, Comprehension, and Production," *Journal of Verbal Learning and Verbal Behavior,* 2, 1963, 121–135.

Frostig, M., Lefever, D. W., and Whittlesley, R. R. B., *Marianne Frostig Developmental Test of Visual Perception,* Palo Alto, California, Consulting Psychologists Press, 1964.

Gesell, A., *Gesell Developmental Schedules,* New York, Psychological Corporation, 1949.

————, and Amatruda, H., *Developmental Diagnosis,* 2nd ed., New York, Paul Hoeber, 1957.

Harris, A. J., *Harris Tests of Lateral Dominance,* New York, Psychological Corporation, 1955.

Kirk, S., McCarthy, J. J., and Kirk, W. D., *Illinois Test of Psycholinguistic Abilities,* rev. ed., Urbana, University of Illinois, 1968.

Kohs, S. C., *Intelligence Measurement,* MacMillan, New York, 1923.

Koppitz, E. M., *The Bender Gestalt Test for Young Children,* New York, Grune and Stratton, 1964.

Lee, L. L., "A Screening Test for Syntax Development," *Journal of Speech and Hearing Disorders,* 25, 1970, 103–112.

————, *Northwestern Syntax Screening Test,* Evanston, Illinois, Northwestern University, 1969.

Leiter, R. G., *Leiter International Performance Scale,* Washington, D. C., Psychological Service Center, 1948.

McDonald, E., *A Deep Test of Articulation,* Pittsburgh, Stanwix House, 1964.

Mecham, M. J., *Verbal Language Developmental Scale*, Minneapolis, American Guidance Service, 1959.

——, and Jex, J. L., *Picture Speech Discrimination Test*, Provo, Utah, Brigham Young University Press, 1962.

Menyuk, P., "A Preliminary Evaluation of Grammatical Capacity in Children," *Journal of Verbal Learning and Verbal Behavior*, 2, 1963, 429–439.

Porteus, S. D., *Porteus Maze Tests*, Vineland Revision, New York, Psychological Corporation, 1965.

Pronovost, W., and Dumbleton, D., *Boston University Speech·Sound Discrimination Test*, Boston, Boston University, 1955.

Raven, J. C., *Guide to Using Progressive Matrices* (1949), London, Lewis, 1956, rev. 1962.

Stutsman, R., *Merrill-Palmer Scale*, Chicago, Stoelting, 1931.

Templin, M. C., *Certain Language Skills in Children*, Minneapolis, University of Minnesota Press, 1957.

——, and Darley, F. L., *The Templin–Darley Tests of Articulation*, Iowa City, University of Iowa, Bureau of Educational Research and Service, 1960.

Terman, L. M., and Merrill, M. A., *The Stanford–Binet Intelligence Scale*, Form L-M, Boston, Houghton-Mifflin, 1960.

Wechsler, D., *Wechsler Intelligence Scale for Children*, New York, Psychological Corporation, 1949.

——, *Wechsler Preschool and Primary Scale of Intelligence*, New York, Psychological Corporation, 1967.

Wepman, J., *Auditory Discrimination Test*, Chicago, Language Research Associates, 1958.

Wyatt, G. L., *Language Learning and Communication Disorders in Children*, New York, The Free Press, 1969.

Speech-Sound [Phonemic] Processing: A Training Program

A general observation of aphasic children is that they are impaired in the ability to process speech signals (spoken utterances) at the rate at which they are normally produced. Functionally, aphasic children are not able to listen or to make the necessary perceptual distinctions for speech to be intelligible (meaningful) to them.[1] Recent studies at the Institute for Childhood Aphasia (Morehead, Eisenson, and Johnston, 1971; Rosenthal, 1970) support earlier impressions that aphasic children do have difficulty in establishing phonemic dis-

[1]Perceptual problems were considered earlier in Chapter 2. See also Eisenson (1966 and 1968) and McReynolds (1966) for discussion of possible auditory perceptual disturbances in aphasic children.

Chapter 6

criminations as well as in sequencing (processing the correct order) of speech signals at the rate at which such signals normally occur in conversational speech.[2].

Assumptions for Training Program

Our training program in speech-sound processing is based on several assumption that are supported by clinical observations and by some of the investigations indicated above.

1. With rare exception, hearing (the physical reception of sound) is not a significant problem. Excluding those children who may be designated as deaf-aphasic, although some of the children do show mild-to-moderate hearing loss, they can hear normal conversational speech.

2. Discrimination of isolated vowels presents no problem that cannot be dealt with in early training.

3. Consonant sound discrimination difficulty is greatest for fricatives and affricates, next greatest for stops, and least difficult for nasals.

4. Aphasic children have greater difficulty in processing (discriminating between) speech sounds that are different in regard to a single feature or characteristic than where the sounds are different by two or three features.[3]

5. In general, aphasic children require a longer time interval between speech signals for correct processing (discrimination and determination of temporal order) than do normal speaking children.

6. Speech-sound processing is subject to improvement as a result of specific training.[4]

[2]For a discussion of normal phonemic development, see Winitz (1969), chap. 2.

[3]Sound characteristics (distinctive features) may be defined as those aspects of the production of speech sounds that permit a listener to perceive one sound (phoneme) as being different from another. Distinctive features include voicing, place of articulation (articulators most actively involved), nasality, tenseness of articulation, stoppage or maintained flow of air, fricativeness, etc. Chomsky and Halle (1968) present a detailed exposition of the sound patterns of English that incorporate distinctive feature concepts. Winitz (1969, pp. 79–96) discusses the acquisition of speech sounds in relationship to distinctve features.

[4]It is possible that, for some children, the training serves to overcome previously established perceptual defenses against spoken utterance. For others,

APPROACHES FOR SPEECH-SOUND PROCESSING

Environmental Noise Discrimination

In our discussion on establishing representational understanding (Chapter 8) we include approaches for discrimination and association of environmental noises. Aphasic children, unless they also have severe hearing impairment, should have no difficulty with the discrimination and identification (association) of nonspeech environmental noises. However, the approach provides a technique or method that can later be applied for speech-sound processing. It also provides an opportunity for the child to be successful in auditory discrimination tasks and so to be motivated to become involved with other auditory events that may be more difficult for him to process.

Mechanical Noise Discrimination

As an introduction to sound discrimination we would begin with the association (identification) of mechanical noises and their source. Thus, the child should be shown a bell being rung or a tooted horn. After the demonstration, the noise of the object may be produced on a tape recording or made by the clinician with the child's back turned. The child is then directed to make the same noise with one of two objects placed before him. Even if the child points to the correct object, he should be encouraged to make the noise for the pleasure of the accomplished deed.

"Animate" Noise Discrimination

The approach indicated above may be used for "animate" noise discrimination, using toy animals that produce reasonably close approximations of the real thing. Thus, a child can indicate his discrimination between a cat's meowing and a dog's barking, a bird's chirping and a rooster's crowing, a cow's mooing and a lamb's bleating, a lion's roaring and an elephant's trumpeting, etc.

---

it may be a creation of awareness that at the time of training their capacity for processing had improved and they needed to be induced (or seduced) to listen.

Sequential Training

As we indicate in our discussion on representational training, it is important to prepare the child to process a series or sequence of noises. So as soon as the child has learned the game of associating noise with noisemaker, we would introduce training to establish listening to a sequence or series of noises. At this stage the noises may be played back from tapes and the child instructed to point to the appropriate objects or pictures of the objects in order of the sounds they make. We would begin with a two-noise series with a half-second interval between the noises, and then progressively reduce the interval to about one-tenth second.[5] When the child is successful with the processing of two noises, we would increase the task to three, and then to four. When four-noise sequences are correctly processed, we consider the child ready to become involved in applying the techniques he has learned to speech-sound perception.

Consonant–Vowel (CV) vs. Vowel

The basic initial unit for speech-sound discrimination training is the consonant–vowel (CV) combination. This first discrimination task will call for the child to establish a differential response between a consonant–vowel unit and a vowel alone, e.g., [m + a] vs. /ɑ/. The immediate purpose of this task is to direct the child's attention to two units that are somehow different. We do not require the child to produce the units. However, if he does so spontaneously, he informs us not only that he perceives them differently, but that he is capable of producing them according to his perception. We assume that early in their training program, most children in need of auditory training will not be able to produce what they are presented with, and it will be necessary to elicit a nonoral response to determine whether they are making differential responses to the auditory stimuli. We can do this either by teaching the child to associate signals with objects or visual representations (the child is taught to point out the correct association) or by teaching the child to make a Yes or No response (head gesture) for same or different.

[5]If tape-recording equipment is not available, the clinician should practice establishing the intervals for stimulation presentation. The advantage of tape recordings is obvious.

Slobin (1967) describes a well-established approach for testing discrimination with small children.

The general procedure for testing a discrimination with small children is to provide some objects they can discriminate easily, and to give them different names. With small children, the easiest discriminations are between different shapes like triangle and circle, and big differences in size. So make a list of the syllables to be used in the testing, and see to it that every pair tested has a "named object" easily discriminated by a child from the object named by the syllable paired with it. There are three steps in the learning: a) the child learns that there are two different objects; b) the child learns that there will be a reward with only one of the objects at a time, and that he must choose, and c) the actual test, with a choice based on the *name* of the object rather than another one. Example and method: a large triangle is "too"; a small triangle is "tea." Use as rewards trinkets, colored sticky paper, or some other objects which don't readily satiate as do foods. Variation might be a good idea.

The speech signals chosen in the initial stage of training are ones that normal children acquire first in sound production and ones that our investigators indicate are easiest for aphasic children to discriminate. Realistically, even for aphasic children the perception of the vowel or the nasal plus vowel should present no problems that require training. Nevertheless, this is where we begin in order to establish a technique or strategy for listening and to provide opportunity for the child to experience success. In the following, presented phonetically and "orthographically," are some sample units for this experience, which may be presented as nasal plus vowel, followed by vowel, or vowel followed by nasal plus vowel:

[mi]	(me)	[i]	(ee)
[me]	(may)	[e]	(ay)
[mɛ]	(meh)	[ɛ]	(eh)
[mu]	(moo)	[u]	(oo)
[mo]	(moh)	[o]	(oh)
[mɔ]	(maw)	[ɔ]	(aw)
[mʌ]	(muh)	[ʌ]	(uh)

If these units are presented for a Yes or No response, the order should be randomized in a sequence, such as:

[mɑ]	[mɑ]	[mɑ]	[ɑ]
[mɑ]	[mɑ]	[mɑ]	[ɑ]
[mɑ]	[ɑ]	[mɑ]	[mɑ]
[mɑ]	[mɑ]	[mɑ]	[mɑ]

If the child cannot make distinctions when the units are presented at a normal rate of utterance, the following suggestions for presentation should be followed.

1. Present the units with a discernible interval between vowel and consonant (one-tenth to one-quarter second) and about a half-second (interstimulus) interval before presenting the isolated vowel.

2. Repeat, reducing the interstimulus interval to a quarter second or less, and finally to a just discernible pause.

3. When the contrasts are established, present the first units on a single-breath impulse as a vowel–consonant syllable. Allow a half-second interval before presenting the vowel. Repeat, reducing the interstimulus interval to a quarter second and finally to a just discernible pause.

4. Repeat as in 2 and 3 above, replacing /m/ by /n/. If the child has difficulty in these contrasts, repeat as in 1.

Nasal Consonant + Vowel vs. Vowel + Nasal Consonant

At this point we are concerned with having the child become aware of the order or sequence of sounds. Thus, the stimulus items consist of pairs of a vowel and a nasal consonant, or a nasal consonant and a vowel, with only the order of the sounds changed. The surface task is for the child to indicate whether what he receives is the same or different. The stimulus items should be presented in a random order so that the child will not be likely to guess, except by chance, whether a given pair is, in fact the same or different.

The items should be presented initially as two-phoneme syllables. If it appears that the child has difficulty with such presentations, then a just discernible interval may be introduced between

TABLE 4. The Common Phonemes of American-English

Key Word	IPA Symbol	Key Word	IPA Symbol
	CONSONANTS		
*p*it	p	*c*at	æ
*b*ean	b	*h*ot	ɒ or ɑ
*t*in	t		depending upon regional or individual variations
*d*en	d		
*c*ook	k		
*g*et	g	*s*aw	ɔ
*f*ast	f	*o*bey, *sew*	o or ou
*v*an	v	*b*ook	ʊ
*th*in	θ	*b*oon	u
*th*is	ð	*c*ut	ʌ
*s*ea	s	*a*bout	ə
*z*oo	z	*supper*	ɚ
*sh*e	ʃ		by most Americans and ə by many others
*mea*sure	ʒ		
*ch*ick	tʃ		
*j*ack	dʒ	*h*eard	ɝ
*m*e	m		by most Americans and ɜ by many others
*n*o	n		
si*ng*	ŋ		
*l*et	l		DIPHTHONGS
*r*un	r	*s*igh	aɪ
*y*et	j	*n*oise	ɔɪ
*h*at	h	*c*ow	aʊ or ɑʊ
*w*on	w		depending upon individual variations
*wh*at*	ʍ or hw		
	VOWELS	*m*ay	eɪ
*s*ee	i	*t*oe	ou
*s*it	ɪ	*ref*u*se	ɪu or ju
*c*ake	e		depending upon individual variations
*m*et	ɛ		
*ba*lm	ɑ	*u*se	ju
*ma*sk	æ or a		
	depending upon regional or individual variations		

*If distinction is made in pronunciation of words such as *what* and *watt; when* and *wen*.

the phonemes for each pair. If the child succeeds with such presentations, then the pairs should again be presented as syllables, with a slower-than-normal rate of production. Sample sequences follow:

1. [m + vowel], [vowel + m]

[mɑ]	[mɑ]	[ɑm]	[ɑm]
[mɑ]	[ɑm]	[ɑm]	[mɑ]
[mɑ]	[ɑm]	[mɑ]	[mɑ]
[ɑm]	[mɑ]	[ɑm]	[ɑm]
[mu]	[mu]	[mu]	[um]
[mu]	[um]	[um]	[um]
[um]	[um]	[mu]	[mu]
[um]	[mu]	[mu]	[mu]
[mu]	[mu]	[um]	[mu]

The same can be done for combinations of [m + vowel] or [vowel + m] with the vowels /æ/, /ɔ/, /o/, /i/, /e/, /ɛ/, and /ʌ/.

2. [n + vowel] and [vowel + n][6]

Make combinations as in 1 above for these pairs.

Stop Consonants (/k/, /t/, /p/, /g/, /d/, /b/) in Contrast with Nasals

The strategy at this stage is to present sound combinations that are distinctively different by at least two features in syllables that comprise a consonant plus a vowel (CV combination). As we indicated earlier, stop consonants are acquired earlier than fricatives, so that our first contrasts will be between stops plus vowels and nasals plus vowels. The minimum contrast units will be for two-phoneme syllables.

[6]The /ŋ/ will not be used for sequence of sound training at this stage because the sound does not occur as the initial sound of a syllable in English. We are omitting the /ŋ/ to avoid any possibility that the child may carry over any expectation that this sound may be the initial consonant of an English word.

1. [m + vowel] vs. [k + vowel]

If we begin with [mɑ] vs. [kɑ], we have two syllables in which the feature differences for the consonants include place of articulation, voicing, nasality, and duration. Theoretically, and we hope practically, the child should have little difficulty in perceiving the differences (discriminating) between these syllables, or any others that are combinations of the voiceless stop (k + vowel] and the voiced bilabial [m + vowel]. Following are some samples of syllable contrasts which the clinician will present to elicit same or different responses from the child.[7]

| [mɑ] | [kɑ] | [mi] | [ki] | [mo] | [ko] |
| [kɑ] | [mɑ] | [mu] | [ku] | [mɑɪ] | [kɑɪ] |

The same can be done with substitution of other vowels as in sample materials for [m + vowel], [vowel + m].

2. [m + vowel] vs. [t + vowel]

Following the establishment of the above contrasts, we suggest the substitution of /t/ for /k/ so that the basic units for discrimination constitute [m + vowel] vs. [t + vowel]. In combination then we would arrive at units that would include the following:

[mɑ]	[tɑ]	[ti]	[mi]
[mu]	[tu]	[tɛ]	[mɛ]
[mo]	[to]	[te]	[me]
[mɔ]	[tɔ]	[tʌ]	[mʌ]

3. [m + vowel] vs. [p + vowel]

The consonants /m/ and /p/ are both bilabials. Thus, this contrast reduces the feature difference by one since both are articulated in the same place. However, the remaining features are numer-

[7]In the interest of economy of space, we will not present repeated pairs, but merely remind the clinician of the need to randomize the presentations so that the child will not guess same or different on the basis of order of presentation.

ous enough so that the child should have no difficulty in discriminating the syllable combinations. There is a possibility that if a child has been trained to become a careful visual observer, he may assume that he sees what he does not hear, and so confuse the /m/ and /p/ because they are both produced with bilabial activity. If this turns out to be so, we recommend that the child's hand be placed in front of the clinician's mouth for the [pa] and sides of the nose for the [mɑ], so that he can feel as well as see the difference between the consonants.

Sample pairs for contrast include the following.[8]

[mɑ]	[pɑ]	[pɛ]	[mɛ]
[mo]	[po]	[pʌ]	[mʌ]
[me]	[pe]	[pu]	[mu]
[mi]	[pi]	[pɔ]	[mɔ]

4. [m + vowel] vs. [g + vowel]

The /g/ is the sound as in the word *go*.

All the contrast pairs presented above include the feature difference of voicing between the consonants, that is, /m/ is voiced, and /k/, /t/, and /p/ are voiceless. The consonant /g/, like /m/, is voiced. Thus, there is a reduction in one of the distinctive features between the consonants.

Syllable contrast pairs to be presented in keeping with the suggestions for [m + vowel], [vowel + m], and [p + vowel] include the following:

[mɑ]	[gɑ]	[ge]	[me]	[ʌg]	[ʌm]
[mɔ]	[gɔ]	[gɛ]	[mɛ]	[æg]	[æm]
[mo]	[go]	[gʌ]	[mʌ]	[um]	[ug]
[mu]	[gu]	[gæ]	[mæ]	[ɑm]	[ɑg]

[8]We have excluded contrasts in our samples for the vowels /ɪ/, /a/, /ɒ/ and the central vowels /ə/ and /ɜ/ and their variants. The omitted vowels present special problems related either to similarity of production and so acoustic perception—/ɪ/ and /ə/—or regional pronunciation variations—/a/, /ɜ/ and /ɒ/.

5. [m + vowel] vs. [d + vowel]

Syllable contrasts are as immediately above.

6. [m + vowel] vs. [b + vowel]

We now have a further reduction in articulatory features. Both the /m/ and the /b/ are bilabial, and both are voiced. Syllable contrast samples follow:

[mɑ]	[bɑ]	[bi]	[mi]
[mu]	[bu]	[bæ]	[mæ]
[mo]	[bo]	[be]	[me]
[mɔ]	[bɔ]	[bʌ]	[mʌ]

[n + Vowel] vs. [Stop Consonant (/k/, /g/, /p/, /b/, /t/, /d/) + Vowel]

These syllable combinations can be constructed along the lines suggested for the [m + vowel] vs. [stop + vowel] samples. We could reserve the /t/ and /d/ for the last because of the shared common place of production (tip of tongue and upper gum ridge) for the /n/, /t/, and /d/.

At this stage many if not most children who were successful in the previous sound discrimination exercises may find the tasks relatively easy and no longer challenging. We would, therefore, suggest what amounts to a screening test for the [n + vowel] vs. [stop + vowel] to determine whether there is any need for training in discrimination for these combinations. A quick screening test might include the following syllable contrasts:

[nɑ]	[kɑ]	[nʌ]	[gʌ]	[næ]	[tæ]
[ni]	[ki]	[ne]	[ge]	[no]	[to]
[næ]	[pæ]	[nɔ]	[bɔ]	[ne]	[de]
[nɔ]	[pɔ]	[ni]	[bi]	[nu]	[du]

Based on the results of this screening, the clinician can develop practice units specific to the needs of the child. Incidentally, if a child spontaneously produces the sound pairs before indicating his same or different responses, he should be given a special reward in recognition of this accomplishment.

[Nasal + Vowel] vs. [Fricative + Vowel]

The fricative consonants include /f/, /θ/ (th), /s/, /ʃ/ (sh), and their voiced cognates /v/, /ð/, /z/, and /ʒ/ (zh).

As indicated in our discussion immediately above, we would begin with a screening test to determine whether and where specific, training is needed for contrasts with fricative consonants.[9]

[mɑ]	[fɑ]	[mɑ]	[sɑ]	[me]	[ʃe]
[mi]	[fi]	[mi]	[si]	[mɑ]	[ʃɑ]
[mu]	[θu]	[mu]	[su]	[mɔ]	[ʃɔ]
[me]	[θe]	[mo]	[so]	[me]	[ʃe]
[mɔ]	[θɔ]	[mo]	[θo]	[mʌ]	[ʃʌ]
[ma]	[va]	[mi]	[ði]	[mɑ]	[zɑ]
[mi]	[vi]	[mæ]	[ðæ]	[mi]	[zi]
[mu]	[vu]	[mo]	[ðo]	[mu]	[zu]
[mo]	[vo]	[me]	[ðe]	[me]	[ze][10]

Syllables such as the above may be constructed with /n/ substituted for /m/, e.g., [na] [fa], [nu] [vu], [ne] [θe], [no] [zo], etc. We would predict that the contrasts with /n/ are likely to be more difficult than for those with /m/.

[9]We recognize, of course, that even if a child perceives (discriminates correctly) that a combination such as [mɑ] is different from [sɑ], it does not mean that his perception is based on his appreciation of the attributes of the consonants that make for the difference. Only when the child begins to produce the sounds, even though his production may be "defective," can we assume that his discriminations are based on the individual perceptions of the sounds. It follows that if a child is producng the sounds, he is not in need of discrimination training.

[10]The phoneme /ʒ/ (zh) is not included in this screening list because the sound does not occur initially in English words and only rarely in final position. It occurs most frequently in medial position. We do not consider training for contrasts with /ʒ/ necessary at this stage. The clinician may, however, make up syllable contrasts if he so desires.

[Nasal + Vowel] vs. [Affricate + Vowel]

The affricate (stop plus fricative) sounds are [tʃ] (ch) and [dʒ] (dzh).

Again, we recommend determining whether a child needs training in any way for the syllable contrasts that include a nasal and a vowel vs. an affricate and a vowel. Following are some combinations that may be used in a screening procedure. The clinician should randomize the order of the presentations:

[mɑ]	[tʃɑ]	[mɑ]	[dʒɑ]	[no]	[tʃo]	[nɑ]	[dʒɑ]
[mi]	[tʃi]	[mi]	[dʒi]	[ni]	[tʃi]	[ni]	[dʒi]
[mu]	[tʃu]	[mæ]	[dʒæ]	[nɑ]	[tʃɑ]	[nɔ]	[dʒɔ]
[me]	[tʃe]	[me]	[dʒe]	[nʌ]	[tʃʌ]	[nʌ]	[dʒʌ]

Other Consonant–Vowel Contrasts

Up to this point our CV contrasts have included a nasal plus vowel and either a stop or a fricative plus a vowel. Nasality has been a constant feature in the sound-discrimination training. Now the contrasts will be with consonants other than nasals, beginning with consonants that are relatively far apart (two or more features) and moving toward those which are different by only one feature. Table 5 provides a basis for classification of these sounds. In most respects this classification conforms with that of Miller and Nicely (1955).[11]

[Stop + Vowel] and [Fricative + Vowel] e.g., [pɑ] and [sɑ]

Consonant–vowel (CV) combinations such as [pi], [pe], [pɛ], [pæ], [pu], [po], [pɔ], and [pɑ] may be contrasted with CV syllables with an initial fricative. The contrast syllable pairs should have the same vowel, and the element of voicing should be held constant, e.g., [pɑ] [sɑ], [tu] [su], [ki] [ʃi], [bo] [zo], [dɔ] [vɔ], and [gɑ] [ðɑ].

We suggest that the order for contrasts between stop and

11Other classification systems based on distinctive features are reviewed in Winitz (1969, chap. 2), and in Eisenson and Ogilvie (1971, chap. 6). Chomsky and Halle (1968) have a more elaborate distinctive feature classification which we do not consider "practical" for our present purposes.

TABLE 5. Features of Production of Consonants in American-English Speech*

Manner of Articulation	Articulators Used				
	Lips (Bilabial)	Lip–Teeth (Labiodental)	Tongue–Teeth (Linguadental)	Tongue Point–Gum (Lingualveolar)	Tongue–Hard or Soft Palate (Palatal)
Voiceless stops	p			t	k
Voiced stops	b			d	g
Voiceless fricatives	hw (ʍ)	f	θ (th)	s, /ʃ/ (sh)	
Voiced fricatives		v	ð (th)	z, /ʒ/ (zh)	
Nasals (all voiced)	m			n	/ŋ/ (ng)
Vowel-like consonants	w			r, l	j (y), r†

*The features of sound production included in this table are voicing, nasality, affrication, duration, and place of articulation.

†In combinations such as k or g followed by r, the r sound may be produced in this position.

fricative CV syllables follow the order of /s/, /ʃ/, /θ/, /f/ and /p/, /k/, /t/. For combinations with voiced consonants the suggested order is /b/, /g/, /d/ and /z/, /ʒ/, /ð/, /v/. Table 6 presents the consonants that may be combined with vowels for making syllable contrast practice material.

TABLE 6. Contrast Combinations for Stop, Fricative, Affricate, and Semivowels

	Stop	Fricative	Affricate	Semivowels
Voiceless	p k + Vowel t	s ʃ θ + Vowel f	tʃ + Vowel	
Voiced	b g + Vowel d	z ʒ ð + Vowel v	dʒ + Vowel	r, l, w, j + Vowel

Stop and Affricates, e.g., [pɑ] and [tʃɑ]

The affricates [tʃ] and [dʒ] present special problems because they are, as the phonetic symbols for them indicate, combinations of a stop and a fricative. Our suggested order for training in stop vs. affricate contrasts is /p/, /k/, and /t/ with [tʃ] and /b/, /g/, and /d/ with [dʒ]. Thus, we would have CV combinations such as [pɑ], [kɑ], and [tɑ] to contrast with [tʃɑ] and [bɑ], [gɑ], and [dɑ] to contrast with [dʒɑ].

Stop and Vowellike Consonants (Semivowels)

The vowellike consonants or semivowels are the /r/, /l/, /w/, and /j/ (y). Because these are all voiced sounds, our contrast training will be with the voiced stops /b/, /d/, and /g/, and we may have syllable pairs such as the following:

[bɑ]	[rɑ]	[go]	[ro]	[du]	[ru]
[bɑ]	[lɑ]	[go]	[lo]	[du]	[lu]
[bɑ]	[wɑ]	[go]	[wo]	[du]	[wu]
[bɑ]	[jɑ]	[go]	[jo]	[du]	[ju]

Semivowels and Fricative, Affricate Contrasts

The sounds /r/ and /l/ are among the later ones produced proficiently by many children. They are also the sounds that continue to present difficulty for many children beyond seven or eight years of age. A frequent substitution is a sound that approximates /w/. The difficulty children have in the production of /r/ and /l/ is not, however, related to perceptual or discriminative problems for these sounds (Menyuk and Anderson, 1969).

Training at this stage may begin with semivowel and fricative contrasts and then proceed to semivowel vs. affricates. Following are some combinations:

[ri]	[zi]	[lɑ]	[zɑ]	[wi]	[zi]
[re]	[ze]	[li]	[zi]	[we]	[ze]
[rɔ]	[zɔ]	[lo]	[vo]	[wu]	[ðu]
[ru]	[zu]	[læ]	[væ]	[wɑ]	[ðɑ]
[ri]	[dʒi]	[læ]	[dʒæ]	[we]	[dʒe]
[re]	[dʒe]	[lo]	[dʒo]	[wɑ]	[dʒɑ]
[rɑ]	[dʒɑ]	[li]	[dʒi]	[wo]	[dʒo]

A Rationale for Other Sound Contrasts in Phonemic Training

It should be apparent at this point that the possible combinations for speech-sound discrimination are so great in number that neither the effort nor space considerations could be justified to present them. What we shall do now is to provide a rationale for the kinds of phonemic discriminations that an English-speaking child needs to acquire (understand) his language.

Shvachkin's study on the development of phonemic perception in early childhood (see Slobin, 1967) is a basic investigation of receptive discrimination of speech sounds. Shvachkin studied Russian children in the age range between eleven months and one year eleven months for their understanding of words differing by only a single phoneme. On the assumption, which we consider tenable, that phonological discrimination as well as phonological acquisition (production) remains the same regardless of the language the child learns, we can apply Shvachkin's observations to children exposed to English.[12]

If we apply Shvachkin's observations and Jakobson's implication to a child exposed to English, the following adaptation for phonological discrimination would pertain for consonants:

Pattern of Phonemic Development (Distinctions)

1. The presence or absence of consonants in syllables: [bɑk] and [ɑk], [vek] and [ek].
2. Stop and fricative sounds with sonorants (nasals, vowellike consonants): *b–m, d–r, g–n, v–y* /j/.
3. Nasal and liquid sounds: *m–l, m–r, n–l, n–r, n–y, m–y*.
4. Intranasal distinctions: *m–n*.
5. Intraliquid distinctions: *l–r*.
6. Fricative and nonfricative: *z–m, v–n*.
7. Labial and nonlabial: *b–d, v–z*.
8. Stop and fricative: *b–v, d–z, k–f*.
9. Lingual and velar: *d–g, t–k*.
10. Voiceless and voiced cognates: *p–b, t–d, k–g, f–v, s–z*.
11. Blade and groove sibilants: s–sh /ʃ/, z–zh /ʒ/.
12. Liquid and glide: *r–y, l–y*.

Our order of presentation thus far has, in general but not in every instance, been consistent with the pattern of phonemic development indicated above. Our order has tried to reconcile Shvachkin's sequence with observations on number of distinctive phonemic features aphasic children seem to require to discriminate between speech sounds.

Consonant–Vowel–Consonant (CVC) with the Same Consonant in the First and Third Positions, e.g., [mam] and [pip]

Our purpose at this stage is to increase the length of syllable presented to the child in consonant–vowel–consonant units using

[12]Jakobson (1968, p. 46) states unequivocally: "Whether it is a question of French or Scandinavian children, of English or Slavic, of Indian or German, or of Estonian, Dutch or Japanese children, every description based on careful observation repeatedly confirms the striking fact that the relative chronological order of phonological acquisitions remains everywhere and at all times the same."

the same consonant in the first and third position of the syllable. The syllable contrasts may be those previously presented for the [nasal + vowel] vs. [stop + vowel], [fricative + vowel], and [affricate + vowel] exercises with the addition of a repeated consonant to produce a CVC unit. Thus, we might have syllables such as the following:

[mim]	[dɑd]	[pup]	[fɑf]
[mem]	[kik]	[sæs]	[vov]
[nɑn]	[kek]	[sas]	[vev]
[nun]	[gʌg]	[ziz]	[tʃʌtʃ]
[tut]	[gɑg]	[zuz]	[dʒadʒ]
[tɑt]	[pip]	[fif]	[θɑθ]

Syllables such as those presented above may be presented in contrast with [nasal + vowel + nasal] or in reduplicated presentations for same or different responses. The intervals between syllable presentations (interstimulus intervals) should at first be clearly discernible—approximately a quarter of a second—and then reduced to where they are just discernible. Finally, they should be presented as if they were equally stressed syllables of a two-syllable utterance, e.g., [mam mam], [mam tat], [tat tat], etc., *with different initial sounds for stop–fricative contrasts* as follows:

[bik]	[sik]	[dʌd]	[vʌd]
[bek]	[sek]	[dɑk]	[vɑk]
[kup]	[fup]	[kɪp]	[vɪp]
[pet]	[set]	[pɑz]	[zɑz]
[pɔt]	[sɔt]	[tut]	[θut]

The list that follows features CVC syllables with different third sounds.

[pik]	[pim]	[sap]	[san]
[pek]	[pez]	[sɔm]	[sɔk]
[bɑf]	[bɑʃ]	[tʃek]	[tʃef]
[tup]	[tuz]	[zup]	[zun]

When it becomes evident that the child can make the discriminations, or can process same and different sound sequences even when they are presented as if they were two-syllable utterances, he is ready for the next step in training.[13]

Bisyllables Differing in Vowels (Strong and Weak Vowels)

Weak vowels in unstressed syllables is a feature of spoken English. Thus, either the vowel schwa /ə/ or /ɪ/ is likely to be present in words of two or more syllables. The need for children exposed to English to "tune in" on the vowel difference and on the stress patterns and prosody of English utterance should be apparent. Following are some two-syllable nonsense combinations that may be used as model forms for practice in a same or different procedure, or in any other procedure in which the child indicates his awareness of vowel or syllable stress difference.

First Syllable Stress		Second Syllable Stress		First Syllable Stress		Second Syllable Stress	
[mi	pɪm]	[mɪ	pim]	[ti	sɪt]	[tɪ	sit]
[me	kɪm]	[mɪ	kem]	[te	sɪt]	[tɪ	set]
[mu	səm]	[mə	sum]	[pɑ	ʃəp]	[pə	ʃap]
[mo	ʃəm]	[mə	ʃom]	[pɛ	rəp]	[pə	rɛp]
[nɑ	rən]	[nə	rɑn]	[su	kət]	[sə	kut]
[tɑ	sək]	[tə	sɑk]	[sɑ	kət]	[sə	kɑt]
[pɑ	ʃək]	[pə	ʃɑk]	[ru	mət]	[rə	mut]
[mu	rət]	[mə	rut]	[lɔ	pət]	[lə	pot]
[so	pət]	[sə	pot]	[tʃa	məp]	[tʃə	mɑp]

[13]If the clinician feels intuitively that the child can process the two-syllable presentations, then these should be presented first. If the child is successful, there is no need to present the CVC units with discernible interstimulus intervals.

Discrimination of "Medial" Sounds in Bisyllabic Context

Moving in the direction of contexts that approximate real words, we would now introduce bisyllables with a weak-strong vowel construction that differ by only a medial sound, e.g., [hə mɑk] and [hə ʒɑk].[14]

At this point we would look for any evident difficulties for responses when the medial sounds are close together in regard to distinctive features, e.g., [hə sɑk] and [ha ʃak], or [hə sɑk] and [hə zak], and emphasize training to overcome discriminatory weaknesses. The constructions that follow are in approximate order (greatest number to fewest) relative to distinctive sound features.

[hə] + CVC Constructions				Sound Contrasts for First Sound of Stressed Syllable			
[hə][15]	[mɑk]	[hə]	[ʒɑk]	[hə]	[ʃʌp]	[hə]	[dʌp]
	[mɑk]		[gɑk]		[dʒab]		[θab]
	[muk]		[suk]		[dʒeb]		[veb]
	[pɑk]		[ʒɑk]		[vɑk]		[ʃɑk]
	[bik]		[ʃik]		[fub]		[sub]
	[mɑg]		[θɑg]		[set]		[ʃet]
	[nup]		[pup]		[feb]		[veb]
	[nep]		[tʃep]		[nup]		[mup]
	[nuk]		[vuk]		[tɑk]		[dɑk]
	[bek]		[zek]		[kep]		[gep]
	[sɑp]		[bɑp]		[sɑp]		[zɑp]
	[sip]		[pip]		[pun]		[bun]
	[zup]		[tup]		[tʌm]		[dʌm]

[14]These are the basic constructions used by McReynolds (1966) in her study. McReynolds found that with training, aphasic children can make discriminatory responses to such syllables, but at a slower rate than normal controls.

[15]The first syllable for each member of each pair is [hə].

Position (Sound) Sequencing

One of the underlying difficulties in the auditory processing of aphasic children is for sequencing (for keeping in mind the order of events) so that a word such as *ten* can be distinguished from *net,* or *pats* from *past.* In early language acquisition, sequencing difficulties are common when children begin to use polysyllabic words. Characteristic transpositions such as *aminal* for *animal* and *pasghetti* for *spaghetti* are often maintained for a considerable time. Our concern at this time is not with production, but with reception and perception. Thus, the material presented will not require the child to reproduce a sequence, but to recognize and indicate whether the sequences are the same or different. Of course, if the child spontaneously produces the sequences correctly, we may assume that he has received and processed them as they were presented to him. In the lists that follow we shall present the syllables orthographically and will not be concerned that many of the syllables are real rather than nonsense words.

We suggest at the outset that the child be given a few items for screening purposes to determine whether quantity (number of phonemes) rather than order, per se, is a basic problem.

Screening Items

kip	pick	pot	top	pats	past
nub	bun	sub	bus	muts	must
nib	pin	lease	seal	nets	nest
bud	dub	stone	notes	claps	clasp

CVC Sample Items for Sequencing

nap	pan	feel	leaf	lag	gal
gun	nug	can	nack	lane	nail
cup	puck	neat	teen	mode	dome
kit	tick	meat	team	pal	lap
bad	dab	face	safe	tack	cat
moon	noom	side	dice	cut	tuck

ash	ax	rust	ruts	animal	aminal
mast	mats	brisk	bricks	elephant	ephalant
pest	pets	must	muts	spaghetti	pasghetti
clasp	claps	nest	nets	telephone	tephelone

Summary

The materials in this chapter on speech-sound processing are intended to provide procedures and samples for training children with difficulties in auditory discrimination. We have taken the position that a basic training program should start where the child is in regard to his phonemic perceptual functioning and move him along to where he needs to be in order to process contextual speech. Several instruments, described earlier in the chapter on the assessment of nonverbal children, may be used to determine the auditory (speech) discriminative ability of some of the children. However, others may not be able to understand or be trained to take these tests. The clinician then has to exercise clinical judgments and make assessments through training.

The informal programs we presented are based on observations that in normal children there is an order of perceptual phonemic development generally along the lines of distinctive sound features. Aphasic children, as we have indicated, are slower in their phonemic development and require greater perceptual distance for making discriminative judgments than do normal children. Our practice materials followed this principle. The last set of materials is intended to help children who still may need such training in sound sequencing. Children who can make these distinctions should be ready for the programs in language production.

REFERENCES

Chomsky, N., and Halle, M., *The Sound Pattern of English,* New York, Harper and Row, 1968.

Eisenson, J., "Perceptual Disturbances in Children with Central Nervous System Disfunctions and Implications for Language Development," *The British Journal of Disorders of Communication,* 1, 1, 1966, 21–32.

———, "Developmental Aphasia (Dyslogia). A Postulation of a Unitary Concept of the Disorder," *Cortex,* 4, 2, 1968, 184–200.

————, and Ogilvie, M., *Speech Correction in the Schools,* 3rd ed., New York, Macmillan Co., 1971, chaps. 6 and 7.

Jakobson, R., *Child Language, Aphasia and Phonological Universals,* The Hague, Mouton, 1968.

McReynolds, L. K., "Operant Conditioning for Investigating Speech Sound Discrimination in Aphasic Children," *Journal of Speech and Hearing Research,* 9, 4, 1966, 519–528.

Menyuk, P., and Anderson, S., "Children's Identification and Reproduction of /w/, /r/, and /l/," *Journal of Speech and Hearing Research,* 12, 1, March 1969, 39–52.

Miller, G. A., and Nicely, P. E., "An Analysis of Perceptual Confusion Among Some English Consonants," *Journal of the Acoustical Society of America,* 27, 1955, 338–352.

Morehead, D., Eisenson, J., and Johnston, J., Unpublished study, Institute for Childhood Aphasia, Stanford University, Palo Alto, Calif.

Rosenthal, W. S., "Perception of Auditory Temporal Order as a Function of Selected Stimulus Features in a Group of Aphasic Children," Ph.D. dissertation, Stanford University, 1970.

Shvachkin, N., in Smith, F., and Miller, C. A., *The Genesis of Language,* abstracted by Slobin, D. I., Cambridge, Mass., M. I. T. Press, 1966, 381–382.

Slobin, D., ed., *A Field Manual for Cross-Cultural Study of the Aquisition of Communicative Competence,* Berkeley, University of California, 1967.

Winitz, H., *Articulatory Acquisition and Behavior,* New York, Appleton-Century-Crofts, 1969.

Therapeutic Approaches I: The Hyperactive Child

In this chapter we shall consider some of the special problems presented by the hyperactive, nonverbal or severely linguistically retarded child. This child is often referred to as presenting the Strauss syndrome. He was designated by Strauss and Lehtinen (1947, p. 4) as a *brain-injured child* and characterized as follows:

A brain-injured child is a child who before, during, or after birth has received an injury to or suffered an infection of the brain. As a result of such organic impairment, defects of the neuromotor system may be present or absent; however, such a child may show disturbances in perception, thinking, and emotional behavior, either separately or in combination . . . . These disturbances prevent or impede a normal learning process.

Chapter 7

Luria (1961) explains the effects of cerebral (cortical) damage along the following lines. Pathology of the cerebral cortex often produces a derangement or disturbance of the potential equilibrium of the basic nervous patterns. The derangement of equilibrium *may* express itself in one of the following ways.[1]

1. There are disturbances in the process of active inhibition so that the individual suffers from excitatory weakness or hyperexcitability. Thus, an individual is likely to make premature responses.

2. Excitatory responses may be affected "negatively" so that the individual reacts to situations with a diffused inhibitory state of the nerve cells (an effect opposite to that of 1 above). An individual thus affected manifests inertness or torpidity and quick exhaustibility.

3. There is an impairment in the plasticity of the individual's nervous process (difficulty in responding to changing situations). An individual so affected may manifest inertness and perseveration.

Our considerations shall be limited to the child whose perceptual dysfunctions have prevented or seriously impeded the acquisition of language. Behaviorally, the child often presents the following characteristics.

Distractability

The child is overresponsive to environmental stimuli that are not relevant to the situation presented to him for attention and reaction. He is excited or "disturbed" by extraneous events. In effect, by responding to virtually everything in his environment, he fails to make an adequate response to the relevant aspects of a situation.

Motor Disinhibition

This is an aspect of distractability. The child, by virtue of a failure to inhibit responses, overreacts motorically and is inclined to make many premature and inappropriate responses.

[1]We should note the term *may*. We should also make the reservation that not all brain-damaged children manifest the behavioral disturbances that

Disturbances in Figure-Ground Relationships

The child may have difficulty in discerning a figure against what is normally perceived as a background. The child, in contrast to normal age peers, may not be able to organize the elements of a configuration—a tree, a flower, a bird on a branch—into a distinct configurational whole for which the surrounding environment normally constitutes background. It is difficult to separate figure-backbround disturbances from those that arise initially from the child's failure to organize sensory data and perceive a figure which is not completely and "boldly" organized for him. Thus, a broken (incomplete) circle may not be perceived as such, so that no figure emerges against the background.

Perseveration

This is behavioral manifestation that appears to be inconsistent with the child's tendency for distractability. Perseveration is the tendency to maintain a response when it is no longer appropriate to the situation. Thus a response, possibly because of the basic difficulty the child had in initial organization, is maintained despite changing attributes that normally elicit a reorganization and a new response. A brain-injured child who succeeds in perceiving a bowl (picture) on a table may continue to see a bowl when shown a picture of a cup.

Strauss and Kephart (1955, pp. 141–142) explain the psychodynamics of perseveration as follows:

> We can think of this perseverative behavior on the part of the brain-injured child as being a function of his difficulty in structuring his world and his possibilities of response to this world and of his accompanying difficulty in changing and revising such structuring to meet changing conditions of stimulation. Not being able to reconstructure his field, he, as it were, gives up and resorts to the same response which he used last time and which worked and therefore has some chance of working again.

---

feature the behavior of some children. Thus, Eisenberg (1964, p. 62) cautions that "the greatest fallacy of all is the common assumption that there is *a* brain-damage syndrome."

THERAPEUTIC PRINCIPLES AND APPROACHES[2]

Therapy, whether it takes the form of adjunctive medical (drug), environmental control, perceptual training, or behavior modification, shares the basic goal of helping the child develop acceptable and appropriate strategies for coping (learning to deal) with what he must in order to establish symbol (linguistic) behavior. In some instances, we suspect that the child's hyperactivity is maintained as a form of perceptual defense that has its origin in a history of failure, which may have been a manifestation of early implication of brain damage. Such a child may be coping by avoiding; his hyperactivity has become a maintained strategy or device for noninvolvement, even though his neurological mechanism at age three or four may permit responses not possible at any earlier age. By external controls and, where possible and appropriate, by adjunctive drug therapy, by seduction and motivation and by the experience of success on some level possible to the child, he must be helped to change his strategy and to cope ultimately in more normal and acceptable ways. We shall now consider some principles and specifics for helping the child to change his strategy.

Reducing and Controlling Stimulation

Although it is not an easy matter to simplify a child's environment so that "the world will not be too much with him" without making the same world uncomfortably bare for other members of his family, it is possible to exercise some control of part of the environment, Thus, the child's own room may be simply furnished and decorated only enough to avoid "coldness." In a clinical setting, considerably more control may be established. Strauss and Kephart (1955, p. 136) suggest that environments be provided "with as few extraneous stimuli (such as other individuals, attractive pictures on the walls, outside noises, etc.) as possible." In some instances a child and clinician–teacher may work in a small, semidarkened room with a light arranged to illuminate only the material on the desk or table at which the child is sitting. The child then has no choice

[2]Many of the principles and approaches we are about to consider were applied by Cruickshank et al. (1961) in an experimental program with hyperactive school-age children.

but to direct his attention to the selected material. The material itself should be simple, e.g., one figure for a page, or one object at a time for matching or identification with no more than two other objects or pictures.

We have found that once the child learns how to deal with a simple task, it is seldom necessary to maintain such complete control. As soon as possible, therefore, we move the child to a quiet corner of an ordinary room and use a desk designed with two side panels to help keep out extraneous stimuli. The teacher–clinician continues to clear the desk of all material not immediately needed for the task at hand.

Intake Modality

We have found that hyperactive children respond better in initial training when sensory stimuli are limited and restricted to a single modality. Children often reveal their own intake preference by covering their ears the better to see, or closing their eyes the better to hear. Intake modality of choice can be determined by testing formally or informally with discrimination tasks. The child who clearly does better with visual than with auditory intake should thus be approached in his early training through the visual modality.[3]

On the other hand, the child who clearly demonstrates preference for the auditory should be approached at the outset with predominantly auditory stimulation. It is obvious, of course, that there are few natural events which make sounds without being visible. We agree with Johnson and Myklebust (1967, p. 24) that "strictly considered, there may be no learning that is *purely* intraneurosensory and it is not our intention to infer that a given type of learning is exclusively auditory or visual. Rather, we view these processes as being at times (in certain instances of learning) *relatively* independent of other psychoneurosensory processes."

However, visual materials—objects, pictures, and written words —may be presented without accompanying auditory stimulation. It is also possible to present recorded sounds without presenting the natural source of these sounds. However, as we indicated above,

---

[3]Based on our observations, this is the stronger and usually preferred modality for most aphasic children.

the assessment profiles of most aphasic children indicate better intake through the visual than the auditory modality. For practical purposes, therefore, initial training is approached predominantly through visual intake. How this is done will be discussed later.[4]

Intensification of Stimulus

As we have indicated, the stimulus item should be simple in design and as large as or larger than life size. For example, at least the first cup used in teaching should be a large, white coffee mug. Pictures, too, should be large and "classically" simple. Auditory stimulation can be slightly intensified through the use of an amplifier. If the room or teaching area has distracting ambient or extraneous noises, then earphones may be used. Earphones serve the double purpose of keeping out extraneous noises and permitting controlled and monitored amplification. Once a response has been established, the loudness level should be reduced to normal-speech loudness.

Selection of Materials

The materials selected for initial training should meet two basic criteria: (1) they should be ones that children are likely to meet in their everyday experience, and (2) they should be simple (classical) and representative (prototypes of the general category) of the class of objects. If such objects can be obtained from the child's home, carryover experience is assured.[5] Inexpensive dishes

[4]Our observations about single modality (intrasensory) intake in early stages of training is supported by investigations of Birch and his associates with frankly brain-damaged children. Birch and Belmont (1965) found that when given a choice, brain-injured children preferred to use unisensory information (visual-visual) rather than multisensory information (visual-auditory) as bases for making judgments and organizing behavior. In another study, Belmont, Birch, and Karp (1965) found that cerebral damage is associated with marked disturbances in both intersensory and intrasensory integration, but more so for the former (intersensory) than the latter (intrasensory). Other studies of modality integration are reviewed in NINDS, *Central Processing Dysfunctions in Children: A Review of Research,* Monograph no. 9, U.S. Department of Health, Education, and Welfare, 1969, chap. 5.

[5]Our assumption, of course, is that initial training for the hyperactive–aphasic child is on an individual basis.

and table settings—cups, saucers, bowls, knives, forks, spoons, etc. —should be selected for the features which make them unmistakably what they are supposed to be functionally. Thus, the white mug is a better example of a cup than one of contemporary Swedish design, and a fork of the sort used in an inexpensive cafeteria preferable to one used in an elite tea room.

The first selection of materials should, as we have indicated, be chosen because they are within the child's everyday experiences and, if at all possible, related to his present needs. As training progresses, needs may be anticipated, and materials selected consistent with such anticipation.

Conceptual Development

To avoid narrowness and rigidity and to broaden and enhance conceptual development, materials should be varied as the child's early training progresses. However, because many brain-damaged children lack plasticity—have, as we indicated earlier, difficulty in responding to changing situations—we recommend that new materials be changed by the addition of a single feature to the previous material used. Thus, if we began with a lead pencil that was yellow, full length, and with a red eraser, we would change by feature steps to a shorter pencil with the same outer color and eraser, to one with a worn eraser, to one with a different color eraser, to one with a different outer color, to one without an eraser, to one with a round rather than hexagonal body, etc. Similarly, a cup might have a change in simple decoration, color (red or green rather than white), difference in size, difference in shape (from classic mug to teacup), etc. By introducing changes one at a time, the child is not rigidly stimulus-bound to his first object and learns to accept objects according to broader categories. In this way, even though language is not used, categorical concepts can be established.

Awareness of Indications of Distractability and Exhaustability

The child who is successful in his performance is likely to persevere rather than perseverate. However, many children show signs of loss of interest and begin to "look for distraction" if the training situation becomes boring. If this becomes evident, a change of activity is in order. If a child begins to perseverate (to maintain a response that is not appropriate to a situation), then the original situation for which the response was appropriate should be reintroduced so that the elicited response is again appropriate. Then a change of activity is in order.

Length of Direct Teaching Period

Although it is convenient for clinics as well as clinicians to have fixed schedules for therapeutic sessions, in actual practice considerable flexibility needs to be exercised. A fruitful teaching period may vary in length from a very few minutes to a half hour or more. Some children may learn quickly and almost "on the fly" and then be literally unavailable, though physically present, for ten minutes or more. Some children, perhaps responding to the effects of medication, or to lack of sleep, may not be amenable to direct teaching for the better part of an hour and only begin to respond when the clinician is about ready to give up. Thus, it becomes necessary to adjust direct efforts at teaching to the child's attention span, to his "perceptual style," and to evidence that the child is responding and assimilating what he is taught. Some children require and enjoy considerable repetition and opportunity for reinforcement; others quickly become bored and seem able to learn with a minimum of repetition. We also have children whose behavior and capacity for learning varies from session to session, and day to day. The clinician who is teaching the child and not the material needs to be aware of the child's variability. Signs of distractability and indications of exhaustability, which have been discussed above, should serve as guides as to when direct teaching should be stopped and some "play" activity introduced. Such activities might well include applications of what the child has learned, e.g., color or form discrimination in a game or simple form (puzzle) board.

Need for Review and Reassessment

Each clinical teaching period should begin with an assessment of where the child is in regard to the teaching program. A brief review of materials used in the previous session will help to determine where the child is and what he is ready to do for the new session. However, the review should be only as long, or as short, as required to provide the clinician with the necessary insight as to the child's status. Too long a time spent in review may bore and exhaust the child. The clinician who knows his child will also know how to pace his teaching for each session.

Perceptual Defenses

Many children develop perceptual defenses for new learning, especially when past efforts with particular approaches or materials have met with failure. The child who cuts off or cuts out may be exercising perceptual defense. To avoid failure, he may refuse to be engaged. The clinician must guard against the need to have the child put his perceptual defenses into operation. A change to an activity where success may be anticipated should help to engage or reengage the child. This might then be followed by a short period of the activity the child previously avoided and this, in turn, should be followed by previously successful involvement. In time, if the child learns that he can be successful with some or much of what he attempts to do, his defenses against possible failure will be overcome.

ADJUNCTIVE DRUG THERAPY

At the outset we wish to make it clear that the use of a drug in the treatment of a hyperactive child *must be prescribed and closely supervised by a physician*. Reviews of the effects of drugs on the control of hyperactivity and their effects on learning may be found in Millichap (1968). Wolfensberger and Menolascino (1968), Freeman (1966), Eisenberg (1964, p. 64), Knobel (1962), and Office of Child Development Report, (1971). The use of drugs, we must emphasize, is *adjunctive therapy* and not "a magic bullet" or a panacea which might make it possible for a hyperactive child otherwise to behave and learn as a normal child. When effective, drugs reduce a child's hyperactivity and distractability and increase his attention span so that he becomes more amenable to learning than he might otherwise be. Thus, Knobel observes that "despite the effectiveness of . . . Ritalin for the hyperkinetic child, psychosocial therapy combined with the drug multiplies and definitely increases its effectiveness and improves results." Along the same line, Wolfensberger and Menolascino propose that ". . . the experimental variable in the study of purportedly intelligence-enhancing drugs is not the drug itself, but the interaction between drug and experimental stimulation." In effect, then, drugs as adjunctive therapy are intended to enhance the likelihood that a child will perform up to intellectual potential.

In our own experience with children at the Stanford University Institute for Childhood Aphasia, we have found that some hyperactive children make greater gains in perceptual development, in visual sequencing, and in generally sustaining attention than they do during periods when a drug is not administered.[6] The results, on the whole, are sufficiently encouraging for us to consider a drug of choice, selected and its administration supervised by a physician, to be a useful adjunct to other therapeutic approaches in which the child is involved. However, the clinician is cautioned not to confuse a reduction in hyperactive behavior as indicative of increased attention. Some children who are inclined toward hyperactivity may, in fact, do better in individual therapy without drugs, with the techniques for control of attention exercised by a modification of the environment as described earlier in the chapter. Some clinicians report that they find drugs to be useful adjunctives in group sessions to reduce disruptive activity in hyperactive children, but prefer to exercise their own controls in individual therapy.

REFERENCES

Belmont, I., Birch, H. G., and Karp, E., "The Disordering of Intersensory and Intrasensory Integration by Brain Damage," *Journal of Nervous and Mental Diseases*, 141, 1965, 410–418.

Birch, H. G., and Belmont, I, "Auditory-Visual Integration in Brain Damaged and Normal Children," *Developmental Medicine and Child Neurology*, 7, 1965, 135–144.

Cruickshank, W. M., Bentzen, F. A., Ratzeburg, F. H., and Tannhauser, M. T., *A Teaching Method for Brain Injured and Hyperactive Children*, Syracuse, N. Y., Syracuse University Press, 1961.

Eisenberg, L., "Behavioral Manifestations of Cerebral Damage in Childhood" in *Brain Damage in Children*, Birch, H. G., ed., New York, Williams and Wilkins, 1964.

[6]In a pilot study with five aphasic children (Poppen et al. 1969), we found that three showed positive effects of gains in a visual sequencing task and two showed little effect that could be attributed to the drug.

Freeman, R. G., "Drug Effects on Learning in Children," *Journal of Special Education,* 1, 1, 1966, 17–44.

Johnson, D. J., and Myklebust, H. R., *Learning Disabilities,* New York, Grune and Stratton, 1967.

Kirk, S. A., McCarthy, J. J., and Kirk, W. D., *Illinois Test of Psycholinguistic Abilities,* rev. ed., Urbana, University of Illinois Press, 1968.

Knobel, M., "Psychopharmacology for the Hyperkinetic Child," *Archives of General Psychiatry,* 6, 1962, 198–202.

Luria, A. R., *The Role of Speech in the Regulation of Normal and Abnormal Behavior,* New York, Liveright Co., 1961.

Millichap, J. G., "Drugs in Management of Hyperkinetic and Perceptually Handicapped Children," *Journal of the American Medical Association,* 206, 7, 1968, 1527–1530.

NINDS, *Central Processing Dysfunctions in Children: A Review of Research,* Monograph no. 9, U. S. Department of Health, Education, and Welfare, 1969, chap. 5.

Office of Child Development and Office of the Assistant Secretary for Health and Scientific Affairs. "Report of the Conference on the Use of Stimulant Drugs in the Treatment of Behaviorally Disturbed Young School Children, Department of Health, Education, and Welfare, Washington, D.C., January 11–12, 1971.

Poppen, R., Stark, J., Eisenson, J., Forrest, T., and Wertheim, G., "Visual Sequencing Performance in Aphasic Children," *Journal of Speech and Hearing Research,* 12, 2, 1969, 289–300.

Strauss, A. A., and Kephart, N. C., *Psychopathology and Education of the Brain Injured Child,* vol. II, New York, Grune and Stratton, 1955.

———, and Lehtinen, L. E., *Psychopathology and Education of the Brain Injured Child,* New York, Grune and Stratton, 1947.

Wolfensberger, W., and Menolascino, F., "Basic Considerations in Evaluating Ability of Drugs to Stimulate Cognitive Development in Retardates," *American Journal of Mental Deficiency,* 73, 3, 1968, 414–423.

Therapeutic Approaches II: Establishing Representational Behavior

Although there may be some differences in opinion as to whether representational behavior is unique to human beings, there is little question that such behavior is more highly developed in humans than in any other form of life. We accept that the capacity for verbal (oral) representational behavior is human species specific. In this section we will consider an approach to establishing representational behavior in nonverbal children.[1] Our assumption is that though

[1] By nonverbal children we mean those who have no functional language for communicative purposes. Such children may have a few single-word utterances, but for practical purposes are severely limited in their abilities to indicate their needs and wishes or to share their thinking through the use of the verbal system employed by other members of their environment.

Chapter 8

these children hear, they are impaired in their auditory discriminative and sequencing abilities—in their perceptual functioning for
speech—and so cannot establish an oral linguistic system as a basis
for representational-symbolic behavior. Fortunately, as Bruner
(1967) notes, ". . . images . . . can be infused with the properties
of symbolic functioning, as can tool-using involving action."

The "program" we will outline is intended to establish representational behavior through an approach that initially bypasses
the oral modality and then introduces oral–aural (auditory) visual
association for nonspeech events. Through this approach the child
may be induced to listen as well as to hear, and ultimately to
process speech as well as nonspeech.[2]

Level I—Object-to-Object Association[3]

① Matching of Identical Objects

On this level the child is presented with identical objects for
matching. These objects should be selected so that they are life
size and within the child's environmental experience. The object
to be matched should be placed in direct view of the child at a
distance of 12 to 18 inches and the object for the matching immediately in front of the child. The clinician demonstrates that
one object is to be placed next to the other. By pantomime the
child is instructed to imitate the action.[4] If he fails to do this,
then the clinician goes through the action with the child by placing
and holding his hand over the object and moving it to the object
to be matched.

Objects for matching may include pieces of fruit, such as apples
or oranges; cups, saucers, spoons; blocks (wood or plastic), combs,
large buttons, keys, and other items that the child may be expected
to have had exposure to and experience with in his home.

This task is, obviously, an easy one and has as its purpose

[2]The program to be described was originally developed for the hyperactive,
nonverbal child. We believe that it has broader application to other nonverbal
(congenitally aphasic) children.

[3]If it becomes quickly apparent in working with a child that he has no
difficulty with object matching (association), then he should be moved directly
to visual representation (picture) tasks. These are described later.

[4]Successful (correct) performances will be reinforced by an M & M type of
reward or by some form of social approval such as a gentle pat on the back, a
smile, or a nod of approval. We suggest beginning with a quickly edible reward.

the establishment of a procedure—a simple action based on visual stimulation that will be used in the next steps.

The next step is to have the child select one of two objects to be matched with the "target" object. If this step is established, then the assortment of objects available for selection may be increased from two to three.

We have found that some children will not perform the task required if the object to be matched is not placed within an enclosed field or structure. Some children will reject the task of placing one object next to another on an open surface, but will perform correctly if the target object is in an enclosure such as an open wood or cardboard box large enough to receive a second "like object."

We recommend that, at first, the selection material contain the like object and one unlike object, e.g., a spoon and a block of wood for matching to a spoon. In a later step, related objects, e.g., a cup and a spoon, plus an unrelated one such as a comb, may be used to match with a cup.

2. Matching of Like-but-Not-Identical Objects

This step is intended to establish the notion of near-likenesses despite differences. It is essentially a first step in the development of categorical behavior. The first unlike feature may be one of size, so that the child's task now is to match a small spoon—a teaspoon —with a soup spoon, or a small block with a large block. Then, in keeping with the suggestions presented in Chapter 7 on therapeutic principles and approaches, changes in features of the objects to be matched should be introduced, one feature at a time, until the child is able to appreciate that likenesses are determined by essential features and not by incidental attributes. Ultimately, of course, what we hope to have the child appreciate is that a ball is to bounce or to throw or to catch and that a block is for building, etc. The next step is intended to move the child further toward categorical behavior.

Level II—Categorical Matching

In our discussion on perception (Chapter 2), we indicated that perception is a process of categorization or organization of events into classes or categories. A *category* represents a group of experiences that, despite differences, have common features or a common denominator. The ability to categorize, which is unconsciously and spontaneously arrived at by normal children, is retarded or impaired in brain-damaged children. If the normal acquisition of language (speech) is affected, as it is, of course, with aphasic children, categorization or concept formation is also impeded. Thus, Johnson and Myklebust (1967, p. 44) observe: "In terms of remedial education, experience indicates that the teacher must be aware that some children form concepts spontaneously when they acquire the necessary verbal facility. On the other hand, many must be assisted in learning to generalize and categorize." The program that follows is intended to help the nonverbal child establish categorical behavior on an elementary level. Actually, a first step in this direction was taken in the matching of like-but-not-identical objects described above. This kind of matching may be continued by providing the child with opportunity to match life-size objects to reduced-size (toy-game) objects, such as spoons, plates, etc., made of the same materials, and then with objects made of different materials, e.g., metal and plastic tableware. A further step in the direction of the representational might be to match real pieces of fruit to wax fruit.

Following are some suggested objects that may be used to establish categorical matchings:[5]

Target Grouping	Items for Selection
Knife, fork	Block, spoon
Orange, apple	Banana, button
Cup, plate, bowl	Glass (clear plastic), ball, spool of thread
Paper, pencil	Pen, spoon, button
Orange, apple	Lemon, fork, paper clip
Carrot, potato	Pea pod, pencil, block
Orange, apple, peach (all wax)	Grape bunch (wax), spoon, pencil

[5]Now the target for matching is a group (two or three objects). The object to make the match should be included with one or two other unlike objects for selection by the child. Demonstration by the clinician is in order

Level III—Matching by Associated Function

On this level we are interested in establishing categorization and conceptualization based on associated functions of objects which are basically different in form and physical features. This is the function tested in the Illinois Test of Psycholinguistic Abilities (Kirk, et al., 1968) subtest for visual association in which pictures are used and the child is asked to indicate (select) the appropriate item from a picture card to respond to "What goes with this?"

We suggest beginning with a target object and two from the selection assortment. The clinician should demonstrate the selection and matching procedure and then, by pantomime, direct the child to proceed.

Following are some suggested tasks for association by function:

Item to be Matched	Items for Selection
Cup	Spoon, pencil
Nail	Hammer
Needle	Spool of thread (or piece of black thread)
Paper	Pencil or dark crayon
Lock	Nail, key, comb
Shoe (unlaced)	Lace, spoon
Purse	Coin, nail
Bowl	Soup spoon, pencil
Paper (orange or red)	Scissors, nail

This step may be repeated with a third item added to the selection box.

If the child at this stage begins to indicate some comprehension of spoken language, the instruction may be given verbally, e.g., "Show me which one goes with this."

---

if the child does not initiate the selection, or appears to be making random selection. The clinician may also demonstrate pretended use of the objects.

Items such as those shown above may also be used to have the child demonstrate actual use. However, threading a needle and lacing a shoe should not be included. The child may, though, after demonstration be encouraged to stir a spoon in a cup, put a coin in a purse, indicate the use of a soup spoon in a bowl, and mark a paper with a pencil or crayon.

Visual Representation (Pictures)

The use of three-dimensional objects chosen so that they are within the child's experience imposes obvious restraints and limitations as to the tasks involved to establish categorical matching. The use of pictures widens the selection as well as raises the level of representational functioning. The pictures should at first be in realistic color and life size. The target picture (picture to be matched) should be on a card with a framed border. The selection card should contain two pictures for the first tasks and no more than three items, widely separated, for the later tasks. The first selections should be pictures of items that were used in the object matchings. Later selections may include any picture representations of animate or inanimate items in the child's environment.

After the child has demonstrated ability to match full-size pictures, ones with reduced size (half to quarter size) should be introduced. The first assortment should include realistic color. These should be followed by black-and-white pictures, and finally by line drawings. If the child has difficulty at any of these stages, intermediate steps in which items from one level can be matched with items from the next can be introduced, e.g., a picture to a three-dimensional object, a reduced-size color picture to a full-size picture, a black and white to a color, or a line drawing to a black and white. As review, and to avoid any inclination to the child's becoming stimulus-bound in his matching behavior, the child should be given opportunities for practice along the lines just suggested.

Following are some samples that may be used for picture matching and association:[6]

---

[6]A slot board may be used with most children for the exercises that follow. The target item or items are placed on the highest slot level, and the selection items on the lowest level.

Identical Pictures

Target Picture	Items for Selection
Orange	Orange, block of wood
Apple	Apple, comb
Pencil	Pencil, pea pod
Spoon	Spoon, pencil, carrot
Cup	Cup, knife, comb
Comb	Comb, spoon, pencil
Button	Button, key, block
Saucer	Saucer, comb, orange
Key	Key, nail, pencil
Glass	Glass, cup, apple

Like Pictures

The items above or other common object pictures but with variations as to size, color, and decoration may be used. However, avoid using pictures that are too highly decorated or "busy."

A variation of like pictures may be introduced that show animate beings in different postures, e.g., a cat sitting and a cat lying asleep, a dog standing (walking position) and a dog in "begging" position, a child full face and a child in profile, a boy walking and a boy hopping on one leg.

Categorical Matching

Target Picture	Selection Assortment
Cup	Saucer, block, pencil
Apple	Peach, spoon, crayon
Shoe	Stocking, apple
Cup, saucer	Bowl, comb, key
Pencil, pen	Crayon, spoon, banana
Apple, orange	Peach, knife, key
Paper, envelope	Pencil, spoon, saucer
Potato, carrot	Ear of corn, pencil, ball

Matching by Function

The task now is to associate items that complement one another as to their use. Essentially, if verbalized, it would be to answer the question "Which one do you use with *this?*" *This,* of course, is the target item.

Target Item	Selection for Matching
Lock	Key, comb
Cup	Spoon, apple
Shoe	Sock, block
Hand	Glove or mitten, potato
Nail	Hammer, cup, shoe
Glass	Pitcher with fluid, stocking, block
Shoe	Lace, glove, crayon
Needle	Thread or spool of thread, block, shoe
Paper	Scissors, crayon, cup
Toothbrush	Toothpaste tube, button, key

A variation of categorical matching is to train the child to discern and select the odd item, *the one that does not belong,* in a series presented to him. Thus, items used above may now be presented in a slot board that includes those indicated above for the target item and those from the selection assortment, e.g., apple, orange, peach, block; shoe, sock, hammer, glove; comb, hair brush, glass; cup, nail, saucer, spoon, etc. The clinician must be careful to vary the placement of the odd item in the series so that the child will not make his decision on the basis of position.

Matching of geometric forms may now be introduced using the basic forms of a circle, square, triangle, rectangle, a pentagon, and a hexagon. A first step in this matching, to permit easy handling, may be through the use of three-dimensional figures about one-quarter inch thick. If the child has difficulty in manual manipulation, then further matchings should continue to be with three-dimensional forms. If the child has no manipulative difficulty, then sturdy cardboard cutouts may be used. In training, the child should learn to match any like form, regardless of material, to another like form, with variations introduced as to size and color of form. Finally, matching should be made with pictures of forms on cards or on pages of a manual, with pointing rather than placing as the method.

Categorical training may take place with geometric forms by having the child match two or three target objects from an assortment in a box. If the child finds this confusing, then the clinician may hand the child one form at a time from an inventory under his (the clinician's) control.

Form boards are used to train the child to a different mode of visual perception. The child must now "see" the relationship between the receptacle or well-space for a form and the three-dimensional object. We suggest for the initial step beginning with a single-target form board and two quite different forms, e.g., a circle and a square. We would then introduce a rectangle (circle plus rectangle from selection) and the other forms one at a time for matching against a circle. A further step is to use the same sequence of forms for matching against a different target object, e.g., a square. A final step, which many of the children may not achieve, would be the matching of a pentagon or hexagon with pentagon and hexagon in the selection assortment. In any of the form-board tasks it is acceptable for the child to employ pointing rather than placement to indicate his matching.

If the child has difficulty in initial matching, then a form-board well should be outlined in red or black to provide a clear frame for the target form.

Sequencing

The task in sequencing is for the child to decide "What comes next?" when he is presented with an array of visual events with an established order. Such an order might be wood cubes with alternating top surfaces of red–white–red–white–red . . . or with pictures on the top surface of orange–red apple–orange–red apple. . . . Another procedure, which is employed in the Leiter scale, is to match blocks to a visual strip display. This may be used as a first step and a demonstration teaching approach. However, the ultimate objective is to have the child finish a sequence based on a rule or principle he evolves rather than on a match-to-sample basis.

Plastic chips should replace the use of blocks for children who are able to manipulate the former. We suggest using chips, or sturdy cardboard squares, with pictures of objects, animals, and persons (girl, boy, man, woman; baby, mother, etc.) for the early sequencing tasks. Later sequencing may include the use of the geometric forms: circle, square, triangle, pentagon, hexagon, and a cross. Alternations should at first be for a pattern such as ○ □ ○ □ ○ . . . followed by a pattern such as ○ ○ □ □ ○ ○ □ □ ○ ○ □ □. . . . The items to complete the pattern should at first be limited only to those that are appropriate. In later tasks the selection items may include one or two which would not be appropriate, e.g., fruit chips for a people sequence, or people chips for a geometric series.

Sequencing and Recall

This level of sequencing requires the child to observe an arrangement of stimulus items and to reproduce the arrangement based on recall. The child must now perceive that there is a pattern or arrangement of events and reproduce it based on his memory or inner perception. If a principle is involved, e.g., alternation, the task calls for him to apply the principle to the materials available to him.

The materials used in sequencing may include any of those used in the matching tasks that will maintain their position once put in place. We recommend the use of interesting and meaningful materials for the child rather than abstract or nonsense forms. The reproduction of a three- or four-item series is a reasonable objective. First selection of sequences should include only those items which were used in the presented patterns. Later selections may include one or two inappropriate items so that the child may exercise discriminative ability. If the child becomes confused by the inclusion of nonbelonging items in the selection assortment, these items should be removed.

Visual Sequential Memory is included as a test item in the ITPA battery (Kirk et al., 1968). In the ITPA, chips are used. The stimulus item (sequence) is a card with an arrangement of forms which is exposed to the child for five seconds. After the exposure period the stimulus card is removed, and the child is expected to replicate the exposed sequence by arranging chips on a tray in a corresponding order.

Visual-Auditory Association

Up to this point in our program for the hyperactive, nonverbal child we have bypassed the auditory modality to establish visual perceptual and representational behavior. Through our procedures and materials we intended to provide the child with opportunities to develop strategies for coping (for behaving appropriately) in situations that are within his sensory and perceptual capacities. Our objective at this stage of training for visual-auditory associations is to involve the child in listening, to induce and, if necessary, seduce him in the processing of auditory events so that he can make sense out of sound. This is especially important for the child who has "turned off" sound and has ceased trying to listen even to the nonhuman (nonspeech) sounds which he has the capacity to process.

The next major step in the prelanguage training program is to establish associations between a characteristic sound and the object which is involved in its production. Visual-auditory associations may include animate as well as inanimate objects which, when acted upon, make consistent and identifiable noises.

Noise Producers—"Animate"

Fortunately, many toy animals which can be manipulated to produce sounds (noises) that are close approximations to the real thing are now available. The representational animate objects should at first be limited to sound (noise) producers—human speech not included—in the child's environment. Such a selection might include a cat, dog, bird, and a baby doll. An expanded inventory, depending upon the individual child and his particular extended environment, might include a cow, lamb, zoo animals, rooster, bee, etc. The criteria for selection are the actuality of experience for the child, and the "natural" noise made by the object.

In establishing the association, the clinician should demonstrate how the noise is produced by the manipulation of a toy object. After the demonstration the child is then helped to do the manipulation himself, preferably by direct imitation of the clinician. Then the routine is repeated with a second object. When the noise-producing manipulation is established, the child is presented with two noise producers, and directed to match (point to) the noise produced on tape or by a toy manipulated out of sight by the clinician. Three and finally four "animate" noisemakers may be used in later matchings.

Noise Producers—"Nonanimate"

Doors bang, bells clang, telephones ring, vacuum cleaners whir, horns toot, drums beat, etc. Actually, of course, these objects need to be acted upon to make their characteristic noises. Here, too, our toy manufacturers have made available materials that can be readily employed in clinical training. With procedures modified as necessary along the lines described above, associations can be established between the toy object and its own kind of noise. For most children the success in selecting the object for producing the appropriate noise should be enough reinforcement to keep the visual-auditory association game going.

Picture Representation and Auditory Association

As soon as the child has established his ability to make the appropriate associations between objects and their characteristic noises, pictures should be introduced as substitutes for the objects. The use of pictures widens the scope of possible noisemakers, which might now include food mixers, airplanes, trucks, hammer, and other environmental noisemakers. These noises can be recorded and played on tape. The child's task now becomes that of pointing to one of two, and then one of three or four, pictures for appropriate selection.

Sequential Matching

At this stage the object is to train the child to listen to a series of noises and then, first, manipulate the objects and, later, point to the pictures that correspond to the order of the presented noises.

The first series should be for two noises produced on tape, with clinician manipulation of the noise producer out of the child's sight. The child's selection of noise producers are placed on a table in front of the child. After he has learned to produce a two-noise sequence, the series should be increased to three and finally to four. We recommend immediate material, rewards preferably quickly edible ones, for each success.

Onomatopoetic Word Association—First Words

In a strict sense there are very few, if any, words that actually represent the sounds or noises made by the objects associated with them. There are, however, a number of words which come close enough to the natural sounds or noises to provide a small inventory of first words that have no more than four phonemes, including continuant voiced consonants, that are ordinarily produced with a fair amount of energy. These features make the words dramatic and easily audible. Presumably, also, the phonetic nature of the words should make them easily processible by a child who is beginning to listen.[7]

Our first lexicon for visual-auditory associations includes the words *meow, woof, boom, bang, moo, oink,* and *wha-wha.* The last one is for a baby's crying. We assume that there is no need to indicate appropriate associations for the other onomatopoetic terms. We suggest that each of these words be produced twice for the child, on tape or through object manipulation, as stimulus events for the child's response. As in earlier procedures, the first association may be made with the toy object, and later associations established by associations with pictures.

Spontaneous Sound Production

In any stage of auditory matching, spontaneous attempts on the part of the child to make the noise of the stimulus object should be recognized and encouraged. Especially deserving of reward should be the child's oral efforts at noise imitation. The clinician should accept and reinforce any approximation of the

7We suggest a review at this time of our discussion on the functions of the auditory cortex in the chapter on brain mechanisms and language functioning (chap 3).

stimulus sound. However wide of the mark the approximation may be, spontaneous noise imitation indicates that the child has tuned in to sound and is processing rather than ignoring the audible events in his environment.

Summary

The suggested program for the training of the hyperactive nonverbal child is intended as a guide and not as a prescriptive series of steps to be rigidly followed by a clinician. In a one-to-one relationship, or even in a small group setting, the clinician–teacher is soon able to know how much, as well as how fast and how often, a child needs to be involved in each of the subprograms described. Except possibly for their motivational and interest value, many children are able to move rather quickly from three-dimensional objects to picture representations. Such progress brings the child closer to representational behavior than would long involvement with objects.

We have indicated that our objective for the child is to establish visual perception, on the assumption that the visual modality will be more effective for him than the auditory. Through such perceptual functioning the child is also expected to learn strategies for coping, for knowing what he may be able to do, in relationship to visual events. Though not specifically stated, we also believe that the child acquires a form of inner language, a way of "talking to himself" without words, so that he can relate and transform his experiences into a set of rudimentary visual symbols. In effect, we have suggested a program and procedures that reverse the normal order of the acquisition of language that proceeds, presumably, from sounds, words, spoken language, and aural–oral symbolization to written language for literate persons. Our basic philosophic principle is that the establishment of a representational system and inner language as bases for symbol behavior should not be delayed. Ultimately, we believe that symbol behavior in general, including that dependent on aural–oral functioning, will be more advanced and will progress to a higher level if we begin with the capacities a child has and train to his comparative strengths. To train first to overcome weakness in auditory perceptual functioning in the hope that the child will, through such therapy, begin to make sense out of sound we consider to be wasteful of early effort and productive of frustration. All too often we may enhance the likelihood that the child, already turned off from human speech, may completely withdraw from the world of auditory events and be regarded as autistic. We believe that our philosophy and our program for the hyperactive nonverbal child reduces this possibility.

In closing this discussion we would like to reemphasize that our program is not prescriptive, but rather intended as a guide for clinicians. Only the clinician, working with a child, can readily determine the stage or level of progress (where to go from where the child is) for a given child. Based on responses to this program guide, we have found that some clinicians prefer the following stages or levels in establishing representational understanding as a first major (prelingual) stage for training in representational (symbol) behavior:

1. Identical object matching.
2. Identical picture matching.
3. Matching of identical objects to pictures.
4. Matching of similar objects.
5. Matching of similar pictures.
6. Associated object grouping.
7. Associated picture grouping.
8. Object categories.
9. Picture categories.
10. Which one is different (objects and pictures)?

REFERENCES

Bruner, J. S., "On Cognitive Growth II," in *Studies in Cognitive Growth,* Bruner, J. S., Olver, R. R., Greenfield, P. M., et al., eds., New York, Wiley, 1967.

Johnson, D. J., and Myklebust, H. R., *Learning Disabilities,* New York, Grune and Stratton, 1967.

Kirk, S. A., McCarthy, J. J., and Kirk, W. D., *Illinois Test of Psycholinguistic Abilities,* rev. ed., Urbana, University of Illinois Press, 1968.

Therapeutic Approaches III: Establishing and Developing Language in Congenitally Aphasic Children

by David Ingram and Jon Eisenson

In Chapter 7 we discussed therapeutic approaches for the hyperactive child, and in Chapter 8 we presented principles and techniques for establishing representational behavior as a preliminary to language training. Although the discussion and the suggested instructional programs were directed primarily to the hyperactive, severely linguistically retarded (aphasic) child, they are also applicable to the child who is aphasic but not hyperactive. Our emphasis on the early use of the visual modality is consonant with our basic concept of *verbal behavior as a system* that includes any established (recurrent) pattern of behavior that occurs in association with (as a response to or in anticipation of) an indentifiable event. Such behavior may be oral or visible.

Chapter 9

We shall now consider several assumptions relative to the justification for undertaking direct language training with aphasic children.[1]

Basic Assumptions to Justify Direct Intervention

1. The child has passed the normal critical period of language acquisition and has failed to show appreciable increments in verbal behavior.[2] If we refer to Table 1 on maturational milestones in Chapter I, the period between 24 and 36 months is one during which most children have a great acceleration in vocabulary growth as well as in the establishment of syntax. Because of these "normal" accomplishments we consider 36 months the upper age limit of the critical period for language acquisition.

2. The child is not progressing from single-word utterances to phrases of two or more words. This achievement is normally expected within three or four months after the onset of speech. In regard to correlates of maturational milestones, two-word utterances begin to occur when the child takes his first unaided steps and begins to show evidence of hand preference. In relationship to other aspects of language acquisition, two-word utterances may be expected when a child has a lexical inventory of about 50 words.

A more rigorous test of delay in language acquisition occurs when the child, through training or "natural" acquisition, has established a lexical inventory of 50 words or more, but fails to combine words into utterances of his own. He then may be lacking in creative ability for self-formulation. With training, some children may be taught two- or three-word utterances. However, they are still linguistically retarded if their word strings do not include any

[1]At this point it is important to appreciate that the term *aphasic* refers to children who, though linguistically retarded, nevertheless present a wide array of competences in their language acquisition (verbal behavior). Although most of the children at ages three or four may have been functionally non-verbal, at ages beyond four the great majority have established considerable verbal behavior. They continue, however, to have both decoding and encoding problems, which are manifest in their lexical and syntactic productions. Some children, even beyond ages eight and nine, also continue to have phonemic difficulties.

[2]The concept of critical period implies ". . . a timed unfolding of a certain type of behavior, with a corresponding biologically based period of sensitivity to, or need for, normal supporting stimulation" (L. Kohlberg, 1968, p. 1044).

of their own creation. In brief, children may be regarded as linguistically retarded if their acquisitions are limited to formulations they are specifically taught.

3. The child is able to discriminate speech sounds and speech-sound sequences of at least three phonemes. If not, then training toward that end is in order.

4. The child does not have oral apraxia or dysarthria and is capable of producing, at least on the basis of imitation, at least a consonant–vowel–consonant sequence. If there is evidence of such motor involvements, then the approaches suggested in Chapter 10 should apply.

Underlying Approach for Language Training

Our basic approach to language training for aphasic children follows in broad terms the stages or "levels" of language acquisition in normal children. We do not pretend, however, that we now know enough about normal language acquisition to present a program that in all aspects presumes to follow a model based on normal development. Nevertheless, we believe that the direction and scope of our program is consistent with available knowledge.

Our program is based on helping the child to establish a "grammar," to learn with help and direct instruction how to produce utterances, or to make "strings of words" that are akin to those of the speakers of his environment. These speakers, we appreciate, have acquired their own grammars (their rules for verbal formulations) without knowing on a conscious level how they were learned. They have progressed as children from single-word utterances to two-word utterances or sometimes to three-word utterances without evidence of grammatical markers (tense endings, plural endings, word agreements, etc.). Then, for reasons we cannot presently explain, they began to incorporate evidences of syntactical awareness in their utterances. They learned, in ways still not clear, how to indicate the past and to project the future in verbal formulations, and how to ask questions and indicate negation, both by modification of word forms and by intonational patterns. These are some of the things, normally and unconsciously acquired, that we must try to teach children who have failed to make the acquisitions.

It is, of course, not possible to teach any child all he needs to know to continue in his language acquisition. What we hope to establish is a large enough basis of what we can teach directly to enable the child to continue on his own to be a creative user of language—to formulate sentences from his lexical inventory and grammar that he has never produced before, with confidence that his formulations will be acceptable according to the verbal habits of his community.

Where to Begin Training

First, let us redefine our concept of training or therapy. By training (therapy) we mean providing the child with experiences that evoke language, as well as giving him language stimulation, per se, in a setting structured and controlled by a clinician or teacher. The purposes of direct therapy are to increase the child's opportunity and sensitivity to spoken language, to establish understanding, and to encourage his own productions. We assume that for reasons related to his perceptual limitations, his sensitivities and potential for spontaneous acquisition of language were not properly timed. We agree with the position of Gray and Fygetakis (1968) that

The application of this proposition follows from the assumption that the dysphasic child was initially unable to extract from his normal linguistic environment those significant cues to form his base language structure. This environment in normal situations is complex, ambiguous, filled with distractions, and full of apparent contradictions. Thus, possibly in habilitation if some of these cues were re-presented to him in a highly organized, structured, and controlled environment he could, with the aid of conditioning, acquire the necessary basic and surface language structure and performance.

Training for the aphasic child should begin with a study of where the child is in regard to his language acquisition. The assessment procedures described in Chapter 5 should provide us not only with this information but also with approximations of the child's intellectual potential. The psychological report should also provide some insights into the child's learning style, his perceptual strengths as well as his weaknesses, and his perceptual defenses. We assume also that a language sample has been taken of the child's productive utterances, so that the clinician has fairly detailed knowledge of the extent of the child's vocabulary and the length, type, and complexity of his utterances. With this information at hand, the child may tentatively be considered to fall into one of the following arbitrary groups, based primarily on his mean words per utterance count:

A—0–2 words (primary language level)
I—2–2½ words
II—2½–3 words
III—3–4 words
IV—4–5 words
V—5–6 words[3]

GROUP A

Children in this group may be completely nonverbal or have a vocabulary inventory of up to 50 words. They have, however, shown no appreciable increase in their language acquisition for six months or more and, with rare exception, are at the single-word-utterance stage. For those children who are completely or essentially nonverbal, the program for establishing representational behavior in Chapter 8 is in order. For children who are on the level of *identification language* (see Chapter 1), the goal is to increase the recognition vocabulary and help the child progress to the use of words to bring about events.

. We are not at this stage concerned with the child's articulatory proficiency or accuracy (correctness) of pronunciation. At the outset any consistent and recognizable articulatory product associated with an object or event is acceptable. The objects used for identification should include those common in the child's experience, in his home environment and in the clinical setting, which are useful for him to know. The first objects for identification should be limited to those with no more than three phonemes, e.g., ball, car, dog, cat, cup, or those with syllable duplication or near duplica-

[3]We accept this as the highest level at which we can justify continued direct therapy. Children with utterances of this length almost invariably have sufficient control of syntax as well as of a growing vocabulary so that stimulation in the home environment and at school should be adequate for maintaining improvement in language proficiency.

tion, e.g., mama, papa, daddy, baby, cookie, bunny, and kitty. Other useful words which, at some later stage, the child will appreciate as being related to actions include *up, down, come, go, run, take, give, eat,* and *see.* The word *now* has its own reasons for being useful, especially for a child who produces two-word utterances and can manage "Up now" or "Eat now."

Although our apparent emphasis at this point is on productive language, in effect, comprehension and production go along together. The child who is increasing his identification inventory is also increasing his understanding. The child who progresses to the use of utterances, even though they are limited to single words which make something happen, is increasing his understanding of word meanings as well as his appreciation of the usefulness of oral language as a form of effective behavior.

In the discussion that follows we will present basic constructions (model formulations) and function words and affixes for Levels I through V.

LEVEL I: AVERAGE UTTERANCE RANGE 2.0-2.5 WORDS

Basic Constructions

1. Verb + noun, e.g., eat cookie.

The model formulations comprise a verb (an action word) plus a noun (something related to the action). Following are some examples of acceptable basic formulations to be established:

hit ball	hit nail	hit boy	hit box
kick ball	kick can	kick stick	kick box
throw ball	throw can	throw stick	throw box
eat cookie	eat candy	eat apple	eat pie

Although acceptable productions at this level do not require the child to use function words, the clinician should, at least in initial presentations, include these words if such formulations are "natural" for him. Thus, the clinician might present a picture of a child in the act of kicking the ball and say "Kick the ball" or go through the action with the child he is instructing and accompany the words to the deed by directing the child to do and say, or say and do, "Kick the ball." However, if the child reduces the statement of the action to "Kick ball" and does so also for "Kick can," "Eat pie," etc., these are to be considered acceptable productions.

We are not at this point offering any suggestions as to how, specifically, the clinician will create situations to bring about the use of the basic constructions. General principles for clinical procedures were discussed in Chapter 7. We assume that the clinician will be aware of factors such as attention, motivation, reinforcements, etc. We should like, however, to reemphasize the continuing obligation to help the child to establish formulations that are practical and readily applicable for him, in terms of what the clinician knows about the child in the settings in which the child has to operate. The reader may note the emphasis on visuable formulations that are picturable in the suggested practice materials.

The reader may be interested in an article entitled "Teaching the Aphasic Child" by Stark et al. (1968). This article describes a detailed program of clinical teaching based on establishing comprehension of formulations with an increasing number of lexical items. One of the programs described is especially applicable to children with severe auditory or articulatory impairments. Through the use of this basically visual program it is possible for such children to learn the beginnings of reading and of symbolic-representation behavior through picture matching and sequential picture arrangement.

2. Adjective + noun, e.g., little dog.

big boy	small boy	happy boy
big girl	small girl	happy girl
big house	small house	red house[4]
big truck	small truck	red truck
big doll	small doll	pretty doll
big block	small block	red block
big ball	small ball	red ball

[4]Color as a feature should be determined by the child's ability to identify or at least recognize colors.

3. Possessor + noun, e.g., Tom ball (Tom's ball).[5]

John ball	John dog	John hand
Mary ball	Mary dog	Mary hand
Bobby ball	Bobby dog	Bobby hand
Tom candy	John candy	Tom hand
Tom foot	Mary foot	Bobby foot
Boy cookie	Girl cookie	Tom cookie
Boy box	Girl box	Bobby box

4. Noun + verb, e.g., boy run (boy runs).

The construction noun plus verb is introduced at this level because this is consistent with the acquisition chronology for many normal children. Most children establish the verb plus noun, adjective plus noun, and possessor plus noun constructions before they establish noun plus verb. (See L. Bloom, 1970, pp. 224–225, for a discussion on acquisition order of syntactic constructions.)

man walk	man run	man swim	man jump
dog walk	dog run	dog swim	dog jump
boy walk	boy run	boy swim	boy jump
girl hop	boy hop	Tom hop	Mary hop
man eat	boy eat	dog eat	cat eat
man wash	boy wash	girl wash	Bobby wash

5. Noun + predicate adjective, e.g., boy tall (boy is tall).

ball red	ball big	ball small
car red	car big	car small
apple red	apple big	apple small
book red	book big	book small
truck red	truck big	truck small

[5]The clinician will present the construction as "Tom's ball," but will accept "Tom ball" if this formulation is elicited.

6. *That* + predicate noun, e.g., that ball (that is a ball).

that fish	that pig	that boy
that cat	that apple	that book
that dog	that pie	that cup
that man	that box	that chair
that girl	that cookie	that table

7. Noun + *here, there* (as locatives), e.g., boy here (boy is here); girl there (girl is there).

boy here	boy there	Bobby here
girl here	girl there	Mary here
man here	man there	Bobby here
dog here	dog there	Mary there
kitty here	kitty there	Tom there

Function Words

1. Prepositions
   a. *In* + noun, e.g., in box (in the box).

in house	in truck	in bag	in bowl
in pan	in car	in cup	in box

   b. Verb–preposition–noun, e.g., put in box.

put in cup	put in truck	put in bowl
put in bag	put in pan	put in pot
look in house	look in bag	look in box

   c. Preposition–adjective–noun, e.g., in big truck.

in big box	in small box	in red box
in big house	in small house	in red house
in big cup	in small cup	in red cup
in big truck	in small truck	in red truck

d. Preposition–possessive–noun, e.g., in John truck (in John's truck).

in man truck	in Mary house	in girl box
in boy truck	in Bobby house	in boy box
in Bobby truck	in Tom house	in man box

e. Noun + *here, there,* e.g., ball in there.

doll in there	car in there
doll in here	car in here
box in there	boy in there
box in here	boy in here

f. *That + here, there* (as locatives)

that in there	that in here

2. Pronouns: *it, me, my, I, you*
   a. Verb + *it*

hit it	break it	throw it
kick it	eat it	catch it

b. Verb + *me*

hold me	feed me
wash me	carry me

c. *It* + verb, e.g., it run (it runs).

it go	it come	it jump
it walk	it fall	it wash

d. *I* + verb

I walk	I jump	I catch
I talk	I throw	I swim

e. *My* + noun

my ball	my cat	my cookie
my dog	my wagon	my car

f. *My*–adjective–noun

my big doll	my red ball	my small ball
my big ball	my small doll	my small car
my big car	my small ball	my red car

g. *It* + *here, there* (as locatives)

it here	it there

h. *You* + verb

you walk	you throw	you kick
you jump	you eat	you go

3. Verb + verb particle
a. Verb

fall down	go in
go up	pick up

b. Noun + verb particle

boy fall down	dog fall down	Bobby fall down
girl fall down	doll fall down	Mary fall down
boy go up	boy go in	Bobby go in
girl go up	girl go in	Mary go in

Combinations of previously established formulations

1. Verb–*in*–*it*

go in it	look in it
put in it	jump in it

2. Verb–*in*–adjective–noun

go in big box   jump in big box
put in red box   jump in red box
put in small box   look in red box

3. Verb–*in*–possessor–noun, e.g., go in John house (go in John's house).

put in Bobby box   go in boy truck
put in Mary box   look in Bobby house
go in Tom house   look in girl house

4. Verb–*in*–*my*–noun

go in my house   go in my car   go in my truck
put in my box   put in my house   put in my car

5. Verb–*in*–*here, there*

go in here   look in there   jump in here
go in there   put in here   jump in there
look in here   put in there

6. *I*–verb–particle

I fall down   I dig down
I go up   I walk up
I pick up   I walk down
I jump down

7. *It*–verb–particle

it walk (walks) up   it fall (falls) down
it walk (walks) down   it go (goes) up
it jump (jumps) up   it go (goes) down
it jump (jumps) down

LEVEL II: AVERAGE UTTERANCE RANGE 2.5–3.0 WORDS

Basic Constructions

1. Noun–verb–noun, e.g., girl hit boy (girl hits boy).

boy hit ball	girl hit ball	boy wash face
boy kick ball	girl kick ball	girl wash face
boy throw ball	girl throw ball	Kitty wash face
boy eat cookie	girl eat cookie	boy catch ball

2. Verb–adjective–noun, e.g., hit red ball.

throw big ball	kick big box
throw small ball	kick red box
catch red ball	see small girl
eat big cookie	bounce yellow ball

3. Verb–possessor–noun, e.g., throw John Ball (throw John's ball).

kick Bobby ball	throw John ring
kick John ball	throw Mary ball
eat Tom cookie	see Mary doll
catch Bobby ball	hold Mary doll

Function Words and Affixes

1. *This, that* (demonstratives)

   a. *This, that* + predicate noun, e.g., this baby (this is a baby); that fish (that is a fish).

this ball	this boy	this man
this doll	this girl	this kitty
this car	this box	this wagon
that ball	that boy	that cat
that doll	that girl	that dog
that kitty	that wagon	that baby

b. *This, that* + predicate adjective, e.g., this big (this is big).

this red	this round	this small
this blue	this big	this green

2. Preposition *on*
   a. *on* + noun

on table	on box	on head
on floor	on roof	on foot

   b. Verb–*on*–noun

put on table	put on floor	put on book
put on box	put on roof	put on head

   c. *On*–adjective–noun

on big table	on red roof	on small table
on round table	on red box	on green roof

   d. Noun–verb–*on*–noun

Tom put on table	John put on book
Mary put on box	Bobby sit on chair
baby put on floor	Bobby sit on pony

3. Articles
   a. *a* as one of several objects, e.g., give me a ball.

a box	a cat	a dog
a hat	a chair	a man

   b. *the* as a contrast between objects, e.g., give me the ball (not the box).

the hat	the cat	the dog
the box	the table	the cat

c. Verb–article–noun

get a ball	take a cookie	take a candy
throw a ball	take a flower	take a fish
throw the ball	catch the ball	eat the cookie
throw the box	catch the box	eat the apple

d. Noun–verb–article–noun

boy get a ball	boy eat a cookie
boy throw a ball	Mary see a bird
boy catch the ball	boy hit the ball
boy catch the box	boy hit the box
Tom see the car	Mary see the bird

e. Article–adjective–noun

a red ball	a small boy	a small girl
a big ball	a big boy	a big girl
the red ball	the big box	the big car
the green ball	the small box	the small car
the tall man	the big house	the big bird

4. Inflections
   a. Plurals as a contrast with singular
      (1) Nouns

balls	boys	cars
dogs	girls	airplanes
cats	babies	tables

   (2) Verb–noun,[6] e.g., throw (the) ball

hit ball; hit balls	see bird; see birds	see house; see houses

[6]Emphasis is on the evocation of the verb plus the noun. The formulation, however, should be presented with the appropriate article, e.g., hit the ball or hit a ball, depending on the contextual presentation.

hit stick; hit sticks	see car; see cars	smell flower; smell flowers
feed cat; feed cats	feed dog; feed dogs	hold book; hold books

(3) Noun–verb–(article)–plural noun, e.g., (the) boy eats (the) cookies.[7]

boy eat apples	mother bake cookies
man wear shoes	bird eat worms
boy see cars	girl hold books

b. Progressive Form
   (1) Noun–verb

boy running	bird eating	cat standing
girl walking	boy eating	cat sitting
boy swimming	girl eating	fish swimming
girl swimming	baby crying	bird flying

(2) Noun–verb–noun

boy hitting box	baby drinking milk
boy hitting ball	boy eating cake
mother (mama) baking cookies	girl riding bicycle
man driving car	man kicking ball

Combinations of Previously Established Formulations

1. Noun–verb–in–noun (preposition in)

Tom put in box	Dick see in house
Mary put in box	boy look in window
John jump in box	

[7]The presented formulation might actually be article–noun–verb–article–noun, e.g., the girl eats an apple. At this stage, the initial emphasis should be on establishing comprehension before training for production. This may be

2. Noun–preposition–noun, e.g., boy in box (boy is in the box).

boy in house	ball in box	fish in water
girl in house	car in box	duck in water
car in street	cloud in sky	airplane in sky

3. Verb–preposition–adjective–noun

put in big box	look in little window
put in red box	look in round window
come in big door	jump in big box

4. Verb–preposition–possessor–noun

put in John box	come in Bobby door
look in Tom house	wash in Tom bathroom
ride in John car	ride in Mary wagon

5. Noun–verb–*it*

boy throw it	man kick it
girl hit it	woman kick it

6. Noun–verb–*me*

girl kiss me	baby pat me
mother hold me	

7. *It*–verb–noun

it go home	it kick ball
it hit boy	

---

done by using cards in multiple-choice situations and requiring the child to point to the appropriate card (one of two or one of three). When the clinician is certain that comprehension is established, then training for appropriate production is in order.

8. *I*–verb–noun

I throw ball	I hold doll
I kick ball	I hold hand

9. *You*–verb–noun

you throw ball	you hold doll
you catch ball	you pat baby
you hit ball	you kick box

10. Verb–*my*–noun

hit my ball	hold my doll
kick my ball	hold my hand

11. Progressive verb + plural noun

eating apples	riding bicycles
baking cakes	building blocks
kicking sticks	feeding cats

12. Noun–progressive verb–plural noun (as 11 above with subject noun, e.g., boy eating apples).

girl eating apples	boys pulling ropes
girls baking cakes	girls building blocks
boys riding bicycles	boys feeding cats

13. Progressive verb–article–noun[8]

eating a cookie	picking a flower
eating the cookie	picking the flower
eating a pear	riding a bicycle
eating the pear	riding the bicycle

[8]These constructions may be taught as contrasts, e.g., the difference between eating *a* cookie and eating *the* cookie (picture choice of eating a cookie and eating a pear).

Question Forms

Children ask questions early in their language development. At first, the device for asking a question is the use of a rising inflection (rising intonation), which may be applied to a single-word utterance. Between 18 and 24 months, the device is the use of question (wh-) words such as *what* and *where*. By 36 months the question repertoire of the child is expanded to include asking *how* and *why*. At this age also the child is likely to use word-order inversions to ask Yes and No questions.[9] For reasons that are not yet clear to us, data collected at the Institute for Childhood Aphasia, Stanford University, indicate that aphasic children ask fewer questions than normal children even when the children are matched on the basis of length of utterance (Morehead and Ingram, 1970).

The assumption that aphasic children can be "directly" taught verbal constructions based on model utterances is not tenable for questions. Normally, a presented question is intended to elicit an overt response in the form of an act or a positive statement. Thus, "What do you want?" asked by an adult is intended to elicit an indication of what is wanted. A child may point to something in answer to the question or make a statement, e.g., "Want a cookie."[10]

The matter of eliciting question constructions from aphasic children calls for special techniques and ingenuity on the part of clinician–teachers. One technique we have found productive is to structure a situation that involves the child in an interchange of roles with his clinician. Specifically, the clinician asks a series of questions, each of which evokes an overt response from the child. Thus, "Do you want a candy?" elicits "Yes" or "No" (rarely), and the child is given a candy. When it becomes clear that the child understands the question, the clinician changes places as well as roles with the child, who is then instructed to "Ask me what I want."

[9]For discussions of the development of questions see D. McNeill (1970, pp. 96–102) and R. Brown (1968).

[10]It is of interest to note that children with primary (infantile) autism who do speak typically respond to interrogations by a repetition (echoing) of the presented question.

Puppets may also be used to act out as well as to speak the statements and questions in order to model responses through identification by the child. The clinician will need to use ingenuity to create situations that go beyond the "What do you want?" interchange in order to elicit other questions from the child. Through the use of pictures, such questions as "What will the boy do?" can be evoked. Following are some suggested question constructions presented in adult and acceptable child forms for Level II children. We will present other question constructions for Levels III, IV, and V.

1. *What*
   a. What is (what's) that? (adult form); What that? (acceptable child's form)

      The "What is that (what's that)?" form should be used with a series of objects or pictures to elicit an identification term, e.g., ball, box, wagon, etc.

   b. What does the boy do? (adult form); What boy do? (acceptable child's form)

      Use this form with a variety of subjects, e.g., girl, man, dog, cat, etc., engaged in various activities such as run, eat, climb, etc.

   c. What does the boy read? (adult form); What boy read? (acceptable child's form)

      Use this form with various verbs, e.g., drive, eat, push, hold, etc., to elicit an appropriate nominal term.

   d. What is the boy's name? (adult form): What boy name? (acceptable child's form)

      Use this form to elicit a variety of names.

2. *Where*
   a. Where's that? (adult form); Where that? (acceptable child's form)

      Use to elicit an answer in the form of a preposition plus noun; e.g., Where's that? In (the) box.

b. Where is the girl going? (adult form); Where girl go? (acceptable child's form)

Use as in (a) to elicit answers in forms that include a preposition plus noun; e.g., to the store.

c. Where does the boy run? (adult form); Where boy run? (acceptable child's form)

Use above form with a variety of activities to elicit a location (place) answer. This may be in the form of a preposition plus noun as in "to the playground"or just a noun as "home."

LEVEL III: AVERAGE UTTERANCE RANGE 3.0–4.0 WORDS

Basic Constructions

1. Continue noun–verb–noun.

Article and/or preposition are supplied in presentation, but are not required in child's formulation. However, acknowledge by special approval if articles or prepositions are included. The noun–verb–noun construction was introduced earlier for Level I. It is reintroduced here because it is so basic and provides a formulation for expansions to be presented later. An actual presentation might be "The boy eats a pear."

man touch door	man hit box
girl open box	girl eat cookie
dog eat bone	boy throw ball
girl hold doll	mother feed baby

2. Verb–noun–preposition (*in* or *on*)–noun, e.g., (presented in full form), Put the ball in the box.

put ball in box	hit ball on floor
put ball on box	throw block in air
sit dog in chair	put boy in car
sit dog on box	put bowl on dish

Note: These constructions may also be used to contrast *in* and *on*.

3. Modal (auxiliary) verb + noun, e.g., going to ride (a) bicycle.

going (to) eat food[11]	going (to) drink milk
going (to) play ball	going (to) eat cake
going (to) ride bicycle	going (to) pull wagon

4. Noun–verb–noun–(preposition)–noun

boy put ball in box	dog carry bone in room
girl put ball in box	daddy put baby in car
man throw ball in air	mother put bread on plate
John put dog in wagon	Mary put doll in wagon

5. Noun–copula (form *is* of verb *to be*)–predicate noun

John is boy	daddy is man
Mary is girl	mother (mama) is woman
dog is animal	

6. Demonstrative (*that, this*) –*is*–noun

that is John	this is Mary
that is boy	this is boy
that is girl	this is girl

7. Noun–*is–here, there* (as locatives)

John is there	John is here
Mary is there	Mary is here
dog is there	baby is here

[11]Many children are likely to hear the dialect form *gonna* rather than *going to* in these constructions. From the point of view of establishing language comprehension as well as production, the substitution of *gonna* would therefore be entirely acceptable. In fact, if the clinician ascertains that *gonna* is the form used in the child's environment, it should be considered the preferred form for introducing this modal (auxiliary) verb construction.

8. Noun–*is*–(*in, on*)–noun

dog is in box	girl is on chair
ball is in box	fruit is on table
boy is in house	bird is on roof
man is in car	hat is on head

9. Noun–*is*–predicate adjective, e.g., boy is tall.[12]

dolly is pretty	box is blue
man is tall	baby is small
ball is red	daddy is big

Function Words and Affixes

1. Inflections—Review Level II and add the following for plurals:

put ball in box	gonna (going to) close box
put balls in box	gonna close boxes
put ball in wagon	gonna eat cookie
put balls in wagon	gonna eat cookies
gonna throw ball	gonna ride bike
gonna throw balls	gonna ride bikes

2. Progressive—Review Level II and add auxiliary (*is*):

boy is running	cat is eating
girl is walking	dog is barking
boy is swimming	baby is crying
boy is throwing ball	boy is riding bike
baby is drinking milk	man is driving car
mama is baking cake	girl is jumping rope

---

[12]If the child responds with a contracted form, as many normal children do, e.g., boy's tall, daddy's big, then this form may be substituted for those indicated.

3. Articles *a, the*—Review Level II and add the following:

put the block in box	put a block in the wagon
put a block in box	put a block in a wagon
throw a ball in air	throw a ball in a box
throw the ball in air	throw a ball in the box

4. Conjunctions

boy and girl	see dog and cat
dog and cat	see boy and girl
man and lady	hit ball and stick
box and wagon	see doll and wagon

5. Prepositions *at, to*
   a. Preposition + noun

at school	at party	to school	to party
at home	at store	to home	to store
at airport	at station	to airport	to station

   b. Noun–preposition–noun (object)

boy at school	girl at school
girl at market	boy at playground

   c. Verb–preposition–noun (object)

go to school	go to party
go to store	go to playground

   d. Noun–copula *(is)*–preposition–noun

boy is at school	boy is at airport
girl is at school	girl is at airport
girl is at party	girl is at store
boy is at party	boy is at store

e. Noun–verb–preposition–noun

boy go to school	boy ride to store
girl go to school	girl ride to store
boy go to party	boy run to house
girl go to party	girl run to house

6. Pronouns: *she, he, him, her, they, them*
   a. Pronoun–verb–noun

she throw ball	he throw ball	they drink milk
she eat cookie	he eat cookie	they throw ball
she play piano	he play piano	they play piano

b. Pronoun–verb–pronoun

she hold him	he chase her
she see him	he chase him
she kiss him	he push him
he kiss her	he push her
they chase her	he push them
they chase him	she push them
they chase them	they push them

c. Pronoun–verb (copula *is*)–locative (*here, there*)

she is there	she is here
he is there	he is here

d. Pronoun–verb (copula *is*)–preposition–noun

she is in room	she is at school
he is in room	he is at school
she is in wagon	she is at home
he is in wagon	he is at home

e. Pronoun–modal (auxiliary)–verb–noun

she gonna eat cookie[13]	she gonna close box
she gonna drink milk	she gonna run home
she gonna open door	she gonna kiss doll
he gonna eat cookie	he gonna ride bike
he gonna drink milk	he gonna run home
he gonna open door	he gonna paint box

f. Pronoun–verb–noun–preposition–noun

he put (puts) ball in box	she carry (carries) ball to wagon
she put doll in wagon	he carry dog to wagon
she throw ball in air	she carry box to table
he throw ball in box	he give cookie to girl

g. Pronoun–modal (auxiliary)–verb–noun

they gonna (going to) shut door
they gonna kiss mommy
they gonna throw ball

h. Pronoun–verb–noun–preposition–noun

they carry basket to store
they carry baby to party
they carry ball to playground

Combinations of Previously Established Constructions

1. Noun–modal–verb–preposition–noun

boy gonna (going to) go to store	girl gonna go to school
boy gonna swing at playground	girl gonna buy at store

[13]May be presented with *going to* or *gonna,* depending upon which is current in child's environment, or which child produces in response to modal formulation.

2. Noun–progressive–verb–preposition–noun

    dog is running to boy   boy is reading at school

    mommy is walking to store   man is waiting at bus stop

3. Pronoun–verb–progressive

    she is running   she is sleeping

    he is hopping   he is eating

    she is skipping   they are running

    he is walking   they are swimming

4. Pronoun–verb–plural noun

    she eat (eats) crackers   he has blocks

    he throw balls   she has crayons

    she buy apples   he has books

    he eat cookies   she has dolls

Question Forms[14]

1. Review questions *what* and *where* from previous level with expanded forms as indicated below for "Child's acceptable form."

    a. *What:* Adult form   Child's acceptable form

        What is that?   What('s) that?

        What is the boy doing?   What('s) the boy doing?

        What is the boy reading?   What('s) the boy reading?

        What is the dog's name?   What('s) the dog name?

    b. *Where:* Adult form   Child's acceptable form

        Where's that?   Where's that?

        Where is (Where's) the girl   Where is (Where's) the girl
           going?   going?

[14]See Level II for discussion of techniques for eliciting questions.

2. Introduce Yes or No questions with inverted *is*.
   a. Noun–copula–noun

(Statement)	(Question)
John is (a) boy.	Is John (a) boy?
Mary is (a) girl.	Is Mary (a) girl?
Rover is (a) dog.	Is Rover (a) dog?

   b. Noun–copula–preposition–noun

(Statement)	(Question)
Dog is in box.	Is dog in box?
Ball is in box.	Is ball in box?
Boy is in school.	Is boy in school?

   c. Noun–copula–progressive verb

(Statement)	(Question)
Boy is running.	Is boy running?
Dog is barking.	Is dog barking?
Girl is eating.	Is girl eating?

3. Introduce tag question "OK"; e.g., I put the ball in box, OK?
   Use at first with a series of demonstrated actions to which the appropriate answer (for the demonstration) is Yes. This may be followed by interrogations addressed to the child that essentially ask the child for permission to perform an action. The child may then answer either Yes or No to determine whether or not the action will be performed by the clinician.

LEVEL IV: AVERAGE UTTERANCE RANGE 4.0–5.0 WORDS

Basic Constructions

1. Continue noun–verb–noun (with articles)

The boy hit the ball.	The man close the door.
The woman open the box.	The woman close the box.
The dog eat the bone.	The boy dig the hole.

2. Continue noun–verb–noun–preposition–noun (with articles)

> The boy put a ball in the box.
> The girl put a ball in the box.
> The man threw a ball in the air.
> The dog carry a bone in the basket.
> The mother put the baby in the wagon.
> The mother put the milk in the cup.

3. Noun–verb–adjective–noun (with articles)

> The boy hit the big ball.
> The girl see a red table.
> The man wear a blue shirt.
> The lady eat a big apple.
> The dog eat a big bone.
> The man fix the red car.
> The girl feed the black dog.
> The baby eat the small cookie.

4. Noun–modal–verb–noun

> The man gonna (going to) eat an apple.
> The lady gonna buy a dress.
> The mother gonna kiss the baby.
> The boy gonna throw the ball.
> The man gonna drive the car.
> The boy gonna drink the milk.
> The boy gonna read the book.
> The girl gonna dress the doll.

5. Adjective–noun–verb (with article)

> The big boy run(s).   The little fish swim(s).
> The little girl walk(s).   The funny clown laugh(s).
> The black dog bark(s).   The sad clown cry (cries).

6. Noun–copula verb–noun (with articles)

John is a boy.	That is a boy.
Mary is a girl.	That is a girl.
A dog is an animal.	That is a boy.

7. Noun–copula verb–location noun (with articles)

The dog is in a wagon.	The doll is on the chair.
The ball is in the box.	The food is on the table.
The boy is at school.	The chimney is on the roof.

8. Noun–copula verb–adjective–noun

John is a big boy.	That is a little boy.
Mary is a pretty girl.	That is a pretty girl.
A baby is a small child.	That is a small doll.

Function Words and Affixes

1. Preposition *with*

John go (goes) to school with Mary.
Tom go to school with Bill.
Jane go to school with mommy.
Bob go to school with daddy.
John go to (the) airport with daddy.
Tom go to (the) party with Mary.

2. Pronouns: new forms, *his her, their, we, us;* review *him, her, them*
   a. Introduce *his, her, their*

That is Mary ball.	That is Mary cat.
That is *her* ball.	That is her cat.
That is John ball.	That is John dog.
That is *his* ball.	That is his dog.
That is John(s) cat.	This is Tom(s) wagon.

That is Mary(s) cat.   This is Bob(s) wagon.

That is their cat.   This is their wagon.

b. Review object (*him, her, them*)

The ball hit Mary.	The ball hit Bill.
It hit her.	It hit him.
John push Mary.	Mary push John.
John push her.	She push him.
The ball hit Mary and Bill.	The boy see Mary and Bill.
The ball hit them.	The boy see them.

c. Introduce *we, us*

(1) Pronoun + verb

You and I run.	You and I swim.
We run.	We swim.
You and I laugh.	You and I jump.
We laugh.	We jump.

(2) Noun–verb–*me, you, us*

Mommy kiss me.	Daddy hold me.
Mommy kiss you.	Daddy hold you.
Mommy kiss us.	Daddy hold us.
Kitty see me.	Boy pull me.
Kitty see you.	Boy pull you.
Kitty see us.	Boy pull us.

(3) Pronoun–verb–noun

You and I drink milk.	You and I pull the wagon.
We drink milk.	We pull the wagon.
You and I play ball.	You and I open the door.
We play ball.	We open the door.
I hold the books.	I hit the box.
You hold the books.	You hit the box.
We hold the books.	We hit the box.

3. Copula: *are, am, ('m)*
   a. *Are*
      (1) Noun–copula–verb with progressive affix

The boy is running.	The dog is barking.
The boys are running.	The dogs are barking.
The girl is walking.	The snake is crawling.
The girls are walking.	The snakes are crawling.
The cat is sleeping.	The bird is singing.
The cats are sleeping.	The birds are singing.
The boy is eating.	The girl is sewing.
The boys are eating.	The girls are sewing.

      (2) Demonstrative–copula–predicate noun phrase

This is a cat.	This is a car.
These are cats.	These are cars.
This is a dog.	This is a boy.
These are dogs.	These are boys.
This is a bird.	This is a lady.
These are birds.	These are ladies.

      (3) Noun–copula–predicate adjective

The boy is big.	The ball is red.
The boys are big.	The balls are red.
The baby is little.	The man is tall.
The babies are little.	The men are tall.

   b. *Am, ('m)*
      (1) Pronoun–copula–predicate adjective; article + predicate noun

You are tall.	I am (I'm) little.
You are a boy.	I am (I'm) a girl.
You are happy.	I am (I'm) happy.

(2) Pronoun–copula–verb with progressive affix

You are running.	I am (I'm) running.
You are swimming.	I am (I'm) swimming.
You are eating.	I am (I'm) eating.
You are drinking.	I am (I'm) drinking.

4. Inflections
   a. Present tense marker
      (1) Noun + verb (present affix)

John runs.	The dog eats.	The dog barks.
Mary walks.	The cat sleeps.	The cat meows.
The man smiles.	The fish swims.	The man eats.

      (2) Noun or pronoun–verb–noun

John eats an apple.	Daddy drives a car.
He eats an apple.	He drives a car.
Bob climbs a tree.	Mary eats a cookie.
He climbs a tree.	She eats a cookie.

   b. Genitive (possessive) marker
      (1) Demonstrative–copula–noun with possessive affix–noun

That is John's car.	That is the boy's bike.
That is his car.	That is his bike.
That is Mary's bike.	That is the girl's doll.
That is her bike	That is her doll.

      (2) Pronoun–verb–noun with possessive affix–noun

I see the boy's bike.	He sees the boy's bike.
I see the girl's doll.	He sees the girl's doll.
I see the boy's dogs	He sees the boy's dog.

5. *Have to* and *has to* (*hafta* and *hasta*) used as forms comparable to modals.[15]

a. Noun–*have to* (*hafta*), *has to* (*hasta*)–verb

The boys have to (hafta) run.	The boy has to (hasta) go.
The girls have to jump.	The baby has to cry.
The babies have to eat.	The dog has to bark.
The bird has to fly.	The man has to drive.
The cat has to sleep.	

b. Noun–*has to* (*hasta*), *have to* (*hafta*)–noun

The babies have to (hafta) drink the milk.
The babies have to (hafta) dring the milk.

The boy has to eat the food.
The boys have to push the wagon.

The girl has to hold the doll.
The girls have to hold the dolls.

c. Pronoun–*has to* (*hasta*), *have to* (*hafta*)–verb.

I have to (hafta) leave.	You have to eat.
He has to run.	She has to jump.
We have to play.	They have to play.

d. Pronoun–(*has to, have to*)–verb–noun

He has to (hasta) go home.
I have to (hafta) play ball.
She has to (hasta) drink milk.
You have to push the wagon.

---

[15]Strictly speaking the modal (auxiliary) words are *will, can, may, shall,* and *must.* However, the forms *have to* (*hafta*) and *has to* (*hasta*) are used functionally as modals and so are included at this level.

Many children do not make initial distinctions between *have to* and *has to* (*hafta* and *hasta*). We suggest presenting the grammatically correct full form and accepting whichever form is elicited.

We have to eat food.

They have to read books.

Question Forms[16]

1. Review Yes and No questions of Level III with inverted *is*. Require the use of articles.

John is a boy.	Is John a boy?
The dog is in the box.	Is the dog in the box?
The boy is running.	Is the boy running?

2. *What* used in constructions with expanded grammatical responses. The clinician will need to engage in modeling and role-playing situations to elicit question–responses such as:

What's that?	What is the boy reading?
What is the cat doing?	What is the dog's name?

3. *Where*

Where's that?

Where is the girl going?

Where does the boy run?

4. Introduce inverted questions with modals.

(Statement)	(Question)
John will run.	Will John run?
Mary will eat.	Will Mary eat?
The boy will drive.	Will the boy drive?
The man will drive.	Will the man drive?
The girl will go home.	Will the girl go home?
The boy will see John.	Will the boy see John?
The boy will push Mary.	Will the boy push Mary?

[16]See Level II for discussion of technique for eliciting questions.

5. *Why*

(Statement)	(Question)
The dog bites the girl and she cries.	Why is the girl crying?
The man tickles the boy and the boy laughs.	Why is the boy laughing?
The boy is hungry and eats.	Why is the boy eating?
The girl is thirsty and drinks.	Why is the girl drinking?

6. *How* questions may be asked with an accompanying activity. Pictures may be used to illustrate the activity.

How do you run?	How do you catch?
How do you eat?	How do you climb?

LEVEL V: AVERAGE UTTERANCE RANGE 5.0–6.0 WORDS

Basic Constructions (Review)

1. Continue noun–verb–noun (see previous levels);
   noun–verb–noun–noun (see previous levels);
   noun–verb–adjective–noun (see previous levels)

2. Noun–modal–verb–noun (see previous levels)

3. Modals: new forms *won't, can't, didn't, don't*
   a. Noun–modal–verb

The boy won't go.	The girl won't run.
The boy can't go.	The girl can't run.
The boy didn't go.	The girl didn't run.
The boys don't fall.[17]	The girls don't fall.
The boy doesn't fall.	The girl doesn't fall.

[17]In some dialects the modal *don't* is also used with a singular subject in these constructions.

b. Noun–modal–verb–noun

The baby won't eat the cookie.	The boy won't climb the tree.
The baby can't eat the apple.	The baby can't ride the bike.
The baby didn't drink the milk.	The boy didn't push the wagon.

Function Words and Affixes

1. Prepositions *up, off, out, over, under, near*
   a. Noun–copula–prepositional phrase
      (1) *Up, out*

The boy is up the tree.	John is out the door.
The boy is up the ladder.	Mary is out the window.
The boy is up the chimney.	Tom is out the house.

      (2) *Over, under*

The airplane is over the house.	The ball is under the table.
The airplane is over the trees.	The ball is under the chair.
The airplane is over the town.	The ball is under the desk.

      (3) *Near, off*

The dog is near the boy.	The book is off the table.
The dog is near the girl.	The pillow is off the chair.
The dog is near the house.	The dish is off the shelf.
The cat is near the chair.	The cup is off the dish.

   b. All of the above in constructions that include noun–verb–preposition–noun

The cat climbs up the tree.	The girl goes out the door.
The bird flies over the house.	The ball falls under the table.
The dog runs near the boy.	The dish falls off the shelf.

2. Copula *was;* review *am, is, are*
   a. *Was*

The boy is running.	The girl is walking.
The boy was running.	The girl was walking.
The dog is barking.	The cat is climbing.
The dog was barking.	The cat was climbing.
The boy is laughing.	The man is driving.
The boy was laughing.	The man was driving.
The girl is sad.	The baby is crying.
The girl was sad.	The baby was crying.

   b. Review *am, is, are*

3. Inflections: new—past tense *-ed;* review present, genitive (possessive)[18]
   a. Noun + verb

The boy walks.	The girl walks.	The dog barks.
The boy walked.	The girl walked.	The dog barked.
The snake crawls.	The baby cries.	The boy jumps.
The snake crawled.	The baby cried.	The boy jumped.

4. Pronouns: Review previous levels; teach *our.*

This is his wagon.	This is her doll.
This is our wagon.	This is our doll.
This is his box.	This is his block.
This is our box.	These are our blocks.
This is their house.	This is their car.
This is our house.	This is our car.

[18]After *-ed* is acquired, teach irregulars *went, broke, ran, said,* etc.

5. Relative clause—restrictive (noun–verb–noun–clause)

> The boy sees the ball that's red.
> The girl sees the ball that's blue.
> The boy sees the box that's big.
> The girl sees the doll that's pretty.
> The boy eats the cookie that he likes.
> The girl drinks the milk that she likes.

Question Forms

1. Review *why, how* of previous levels. Review modals.
2. Introduce new modals *won't* and *can't*.

Won't the boy run?	Can't the girl laugh?
Won't the baby eat?	Won't the baby drink the milk?
Can't the boy run?	Can't the bay eat the cereal?

3. Introduce *who*.
   a. *Who–is*–verb

Who is drinking?	Who is pushing?
Who is eating?	Who is jumping?

   b. *Who–is*–verb–noun

Who is drinking milk?	Who is hitting the box?
Who is eating the cookie?	Who is holding the baby?
Who is pushing the wagon?	

   c. *Who–is*–verb–preposition phrase

Who is going to school?	Who is shopping at the store?
Who is sitting on the chair?	Who is sleeping on the floor?

BEYOND LEVEL V

At this point we do not have a sufficient body of information to suggest what additional basic model forms need to be "directly" taught to linguistically retarded children. However, our clinical experience with such children, and especially those whose late onset and slow acquisition of language is severe enough to earn the designation of aphasic, suggests that they continue to need training. Even though the children may be assessed at Level V on the bases of average word per utterance count and syntactical proficiency, they do not perform linguistically as normal Level V children do. The difference becomes apparent in spontaneous discourse. They have the forms, but on a type-token comparison with children who are on the same language level and who are likely to be two to three years younger (approximately age three), they do not use the forms with comparable incidence.

What the language clinician can provide as a supplement to other language experiences in and out of school is structured opportunity for the child to practice what he knows but seems reluctant to use. The child should be observed and assessed for his linguistic limitations, e.g., for his understanding and use of pronouns, inflections, question words, etc. Through techniques such as role playing and small group experiences, the clinician can create situations and motivate the child to use particular linguistic forms comparable in form and incidence to those of children with normal onset and language acquisition. We have guarded optimism that exposure to reading will also enhance the rate of language development.

In time we may expect that children who are linguistically but presumably not mentally retarded even at ages six and seven will somehow have learned more language and more about language than we possibly could have taught them.

REFERENCES

Bloom, L., *Language Development,* Research Monograph no. 59, Cambridge, Mass., M. I. T. Press, 1970.

Brown, R., "The Development of wh Questions in Child Speech," *Journal of Verbal Learning,* 7, 2, 1968, 279–290.

Chomsky, C., *The Acquisition of Syntax in Children From 5 to 10,* Cambridge, Mass., M. I. T. Press, 1969.

Gray, B. B., and Fygetakis, L., "Mediated Language Acquisition For Dysphasic Children," *Behavior Research and Therapy,* 6, 1968, 263–280.

Kohlberg, L., "Early Education: A Cognitive-Developmental View," *Child Development* (Society for Research in Child Development), 39, 4, 1968, 1013–1062.

McNeill, D., *The Acquisition of Language,* New York, Harper and Row, 1970.

Morehead, D., and Ingram, D., "The Development of Base Syntax in Normal and Linguistically Deviant Children," in *Papers and Reports on Child Language Development,* Committee on Linguistics, Stanford University, 1970.

Stark, J., Foster, C., Giddan, J., Gottsleben, R. H., and Wright T., "Teaching the Aphasic Child," *Journal of Exceptional Children,* 35, 2, 1968, 149–154.

The Child With Expressive Disturbances: Oral Apraxia

At the outset of this chapter we should like to restate a position taken earlier to the effect that virtually all children with developmental aphasia are impaired in their speech output because of their underlying difficulty in intake. There are, however, a very small number of children who do seem to understand spoken language but who, nevertheless, are unable to acquire productive language. Such children are occasionally, and we believe erroneously, designated as motor or expressive aphasics. For example, McGinnis (1963, xix) includes them in her basic classifications as belonging to Class I—motor or expressive aphasia and describes the children as (1) having intelligence within normal limits, (2) having normal hearing and

Chapter 10

understanding of language, (3) impaired in their ability to imitate words, and (4) impaired or limited in their ability to imitate speech sounds.

We believe that these children are more appropriately designated as suffering from congenital (articulatory) apraxia.

Oral apraxia may be defined as an inability or a severe impairment in the individual's ability to perform voluntary movements involving muscles of the larynx, pharynx, tongue, lips, palate, and cheeks, although automatic movements of the same musculature appear to be unimpaired.[1]

Oral apraxia, as an accompaniment of aphasic involvement or as a discrete disability, has been well recognized as an adult impairment following cortical damage. In the adult, of course, this impairment is acquired and constitutes an expression of breakdown of previously established normal oral articulatory functioning. In the child it is, in contrast, a failure of normal articulatory activity to become established in the absence of hearing loss or intellectual factors that might otherwise explain the deficit.

The Apraxic Child (Articulatory Apraxia)[2]

The child with congenital oral (articulatory) apraxia, as we indicated earlier, does understand language (speech) and may indicate such understanding by behavior which does not require him to make an oral (verbal) response. In an approximate sense, the oral apraxic child is much like the young child between 12 and 18 months of age who is beginning to understand a considerable amount of the language of his environment, but who has little productive language of his own. The important difference between the young normal child who is acquiring language and the child with congenital oral apraxia is, however, that the former acquires productive language while the latter continues to be impaired. As he grows older, the oral apraxic child becomes frustrated by his productive limitations. In some instances the frustration begins

[1]DeRenzi, E., Pieczuro, A., and Vignolo, L. A. (1966) define oral apraxia as "the inability to perform voluntary movements with the muscles of the larynx, pharynx, tongue, lips and cheeks, although automatic movements of the same muscles are preserved" (*Cortex*, V, 2, 1966, pp. 50–73).

[2]Apraxia refers to very severe impairment—literally, a total disability. *Dyspraxia* refers to a lesser than "very severe" amount of impairment.

to overshadow its underlying cause, and the child may be viewed and designated as emotionally disturbed.

The term *articulatory dyspraxia* is perhaps better and more specific to our problem than oral dyspraxia. Morley and Fox (1969, p. 157) suggest that articulatory dyspraxia may be present when no other oral disability can be detected. Articulatory dyspraxia (apraxia if severe) is restricted to the child's ability to organize and produce the appropriate movements for the production of certain phonemes or sequences of phonemes, and is likely to include those phonemes related to consonant sounds requiring movements of the lips and/or movements of the tongue tip or tongue blade. "The child who has such a disability, in achieving the complex motor coordination required, . . . may have a reduced phonemic vocabulary, may omit those distinctive features which are for him most difficult, and may substitute those which he can produce more easily, or he may omit difficult phonemes entirely."

Background History

In our earlier discussion of the child with oral apraxia, we cited a number of factors which, despite many developmental similarities, nevertheless distinguish him from the normal speaking child. We shall now briefly review some of these similarities and differences that distinguish the child who acquires speech normally and spontaneously from the child with oral (articulatory) apraxia.

Responsiveness to Environmental Sounds

The developmental history of the child with oral apraxia reveals that he is normally responsive to the sounds of his environment—mechanical, animal, *and* human. His orienting movements and postural changes—anticipatory modifications of motor set—are consonant with the ongoing auditory events in the child's milieu. In brief, the child's overt behavior reveals generally acceptable and appropriate auditory discrimination and auditory perception. By the end of the first year or the beginning of the second, the child, if stimulated and given the opportunity, is usually able to play baby games—he can clap hands on cue and perhaps point to parts of his body, as well as interact with an adult in "peek-a-boo" activity. In all except that he is not also a "verbal" imitator, and does not engage in echolalic activity, the child gives his parents little cause for concern that he would not be speaking by 15 to 18 months.

Parental concern may be expressed when the child, at 18 months or later, continues to be productively nonverbal despite obvious gains in speech comprehension. Even then, especially if the child's family history includes some late talking by siblings or other members of the family constellation, the parents may well have been reassured by a pediatrician or a language clinician that all would be well and that the child would probably be talking in a short while. Concern tends to increase when the prediction is not realized by age two and a half or three, especially in those instances where the family constellation provides no evidence of late onset or retarded language development.

Early Oral Activity

In some instances the mother is able to recall that as an infant the child presented problems in feeding. Frequent regurgitation, difficulty in the acceptance of food that required chewing, rejection of semisolid and bulk foods, and lazy chewing are recalled. The child may have continued on liquid and soft foods at an age long after his siblings accepted and enjoyed "chewy" foods. At age five or six, the child is happier with liquids than with chopped foods that require even a minimum of chewing.

Early vocal play is often notably absent or present only in token form. Babbling might be recalled, but lalling (self-sound imitation) and echolalic play are often notably absent. Although the child is neither silent nor an excessive crier, as in some cases of infantile autism, there is comparatively little sound play as we might expect from a child with normal hearing.

Articulatory Activity

Examination of the peripheral speech mechanism often reveals that the child is impaired in executing movements with specific parts of the oral mechanism. Such activities as imitating tongue pointing, lip licking, and tongue wagging (lateral movements) present difficulties. These activities may show improvement if the child is able to imitate them in front of a mirror, especially if the movements can be performed slowly with opportunity for visual cueing. Difficulties tend to increase if rapid movement is expected, or if a series of movements, e.g., tongue followed by lip activity, is required. Difficulties are also likely to be manifest if actual sound production (articulatory behavior) is required. Thus, a child may be able to pantomime slowly the movements for *pee-kee* or *lee-nee,* but will have difficulty in the actual production of the sounds that are a normal product of such lip and tongue activities.

Sequential Activity

The oral apraxic child's predominant difficulty is an impairment in the production of the sequence of movements essential for a unit of utterances. The degree of impairment varies considerably from child to child. With individual exception, severity appears to be negatively related to age. That is, younger children (ages three to four), even with allowances made for normal differences in articulatory proficiency, are generally more impaired than older children (ages above four). In most severe form, the child may not have sufficient control of his organs of articulation to imitate an isolated movement of his tongue or lips. In other instances the child may imitate an isolated movement, but have difficulty in executing a series of two or more movements even though each can be produced separately. Performance tends to break down when the rate of activity is accelerated. Thus, though a child may be able to imitate and maintain a sequence such as *ba—da—ga,* the product may, if the model for imitation is presented more rapidly than at first, become *ba—ga* (omission), or *ba—ba—da* (preseveration and omission), or *ba—ba—ga,* or be compressed into *bada* or presented with transposition as *da—ba* or *ga—ba—da,* etc.

Failures to maintain sequential order are not likely to be associated with any underlying difficulties in auditory perception or auditory sequencing. Most children with oral apraxia who are also of normal intelligence are likely to do as well as their age peers in tests for auditory discrimination, e.g., Wepman's or in any informal matching-to-sample test of a sequence of auditory events, including those for speech sounds, providing that memory span is not taxed beyond expected limits for the age of the child.

By age three or four, when most children are well on their way to becoming syntactically proficient and have a productive vocabulary of about 1000 words, the child with oral apraxia may be struggling to produce intelligible utterances of two or three phonemes. The child is likely to be most proficient with combinations of readily visible labial (lip) plus vowel sounds. Thus, he may be successful with *m, n, b,* or *p* plus a vowel. So, he may produce *ma* and *moo* correctly. He may have most vowel sounds under fairly good control. If, therefore, he attempts an utterance with such sounds, and if the intonation contour is appropriate as it is fortunately likely to be, his utterance may suggest the speech attempts of a child who is just beginning to combine words into a two-word utterance. In effect, he will sound infantile. Nonvisible sounds and attempts at sequences of five or six phonemes may reveal distortions and sound transpositions, again suggesting the efforts of a child of between 15 and 18 months, or a slower child of about two years. Syntactical (grammatical) markers are, of course, almost always absent.

Aphasia and Oral Apraxia

It is unhappily possible for a child to be orally apraxic and congenitally aphasic. In such a case the child will suffer from failure to make adequate sense out of speech sounds and will also be impaired in the production of the limited amount of language he does understand. In the absence of intake, there will be, of course, little motivation for output except for emotional expression. The aphasic-orally apraxic child is one who is essentially perceptually deaf for speech and impaired in his motor capacity for communicating what he understands of nonspeech environmental auditory events. In essence, he is reduced to living in a visual world. If we recognize this as a reality situation, and train the child on a visual-visual basis, then some representational appreciation and some language behavior can be established to serve as a basis for future training in auditory speech perception and oral language production.

Related Evidence of Dyspraxia

Clinical histories reveal that many orally apraxic children present findings that suggest some degree of overall dyspraxia. Some of the children are conspicuously awkward, their early developmental histories include late walking (past two years of age) and a severe lack of manual dexterity. Handedness and other indications of laterality preference may not yet be established at age five. Essentially, some of the children may best be designated as ambi-nonlateral, slow, and awkward in all forms of motor expression. A clinical impression about some of the children is that they seem capable of stumbling over a chalk line. McGinnis (1963, p. 36) describes a child with motor aphasia and normal intelligence in a manner which we believe is almost typical of a majority of children we designate as orally apraxic.

There was delay in all physical development. He was nearly two years old before he began to walk, and then needed physical therapy to improve control of his feet and leg muscles. The parents reported that he made an attempt to say "daddy" at the age of two, but at five he had made no gain in acquiring intelligible speech. He made few attempts to talk, even though his hearing and comprehension of speech were good.

Expressive Impairments of the Congenitally Aphasic Child

The congenitally aphasic child without dyspraxic involvements may have no functional language or, depending upon degree of severity and age, may have a vocabulary limited to a few words that may be used appropriately, with specific meanings communicated and enhanced through the use of gesture. Some children may develop a fairly elaborate gesture system, with vocalization employed essentially as an attention device to engage another person in a communicative interchange. As the child begins to acquire speech, later and more slowly than his age peers, his productive language is likely to consist largely of nouns and verbs, or words that serve verb functions. He appears, in effect, to be fixed at the single- or two-word-utterance stage in his language acquisition for a considerably longer period of time than the normal child. Like the normal child, receptive language development is considerably greater than productive language. Unlike the normal child, the one with congenital aphasia has a greater disproportion of language he understands to language he can produce.

Syntax develops slowly, even with direct training. Thus, the aphasic child builds up a much larger inventory of single-word utterances before progressing to two-word asyntactic formulations. Two-word utterances may continue to be asyntactic (an absence of functional words and inflectional markers) long after the normal child has begun to use conventional sentences. When the aphasic child attempts syntactic formulations, he sometimes appears to be suffering from anomia, apparently hunting for the word he needs for his utterance to be conventional and acceptable. We believe that the appearance of anomic difficulty is really an indication that he is striving, however belatedly, to express himself in a sentence unit, that he is working out a complete verbal formulation and is no longer satisfied with asyntactic utterance. In this stage the child's utterances may suggest the repetitions and hesitations of the normal dysfluencies of the three-year-old child, or even the excessive dysfluencies of the primary stutterer.

Therapeutic approaches for the congenitally aphasic child are considered in Chapters 7, 8, and 9.

THERAPY FOR ORAL APRAXIA

The objective in the treatment of the child with oral apraxia is, of course, to establish the ability to produce a sequence of voluntary movements essential for intelligible utterance. The corollary of this objective is to extinguish (discourage) "random" oral movements, which produce the effect of jargon or gibberish as well as some of the perseverative articulatory products that sometimes seem to burst at and overwhelm a would-be listener. A related goal is to discourage a child who has control of a few appropriate, short utterances to "surround" and incorporate them into a larger flow of jargon.[3]

Establishing Sounds in Isolation

If we consider the orally apraxic child as one whose impairment is in articulatory production and not in auditory perception or speech comprehension, we may then take advantage of capacities implied in this designation in our therapeutic efforts. The capacities are for normal auditory as well as visual intake, and so for the sequencing of speech events. We may assume that visual stimulation is associated with the auditory and this, in turn, with articulation. Since even a single sound is a product of a synergy (series)

---

[3]McGinnis (1963, p. 42) refers to this unintelligible flow as "scribble speech."

of related movements, the basis for sequencing is established even when we are dealing with an isolated sound or, preferably, a consonant followed by a vowel. We recommend the following general approach in the initial phonetic–phonemic training.[4]

1. With clinician and child facing a mirror, the clinician slowly pantomimes the articulation for [pɑ] The child is directed to imitate the movements. If the child does not succeed after several trials, the movements should be broken up (separated) into distinct [p] . . . [ɑ]. When this is achieved, the interval between the separate movements should be reduced until the combination [pɑ] is produced as a continuous articulatory effort. If the two-phoneme sequence or two-phoneme succession is not possible, then the child should be trained to imitate a single, isolated sound. If mirror imitation does not result in successful imitation, then the therapist should feel free to place the articulators in position by manual manipulation, the use of a tongue depressor (spatula), a rounded probe stick, or the manipulation of the child's fingers to the appropriate articulatory position. As soon as possible, however, the visual stimulus alone, and then visual recall, should constitute the basis for imitation. Ultimately, of course, the auditory stimulus should replace all of the other stimuli. In some instances it may be helpful to photograph the child's face in appropriate articulatory states. Then the child is, in fact as well as in effect, imitating himself. Videotape playbacks, if available, provide an ideal though expensive apparatus and medium for early training.

The first isolated sounds should be the /m/, the second the /p/ or /b/. We would then recommend the /k/, /g/, and /n/ in that order, followed by the /t/ and /d/ and /l/ and /r/. The sibilant sounds, /s/, /z/, /ʃ/, and /ʒ/ should follow, and finally the

[4]McGinnis (1963, pp. 134–137), describes a series of initial training steps under the heading "development of the elements of speech." These are exercises for "gross" tongue movements and tongue position (tongue protrusion, tongue pointing, tongue clicking) which may be performed in an individual or group situation. McGinnis, it should be noted, recommends that a mirror should not be used in training a child to imitate gross muscle patterns. "Unless there is extreme difficulty in tongue control the child should be able to imitate tongue movements from the pattern given by the teacher" (p. 135). Other procedures are described by McGinnis for training an apraxic child (pp. 81–88). The essentials of the motokinesthetic (Young and Hawk, 1955) are also appropriate for the establishment of isolated speech sounds and for sound sequences.

/θ/ and/ð/. However, if the child produces a /θ/ or /ð/ as a substitution (approximation) for one of the other sounds, we would establish the child's product on a voluntary and appropriate basis by training him to imitate these sounds on an imitative basis.[5]

2. Repeat as above, but this time without the use of a mirror and with the child facing the clinician.

3. Direct the child to produce the movements with his eyes closed, so that visual memory becomes the basis for recall.

4. Introduce vocalization so that the child now hears and sees the activity producing the contexts [pɑ] and [bɑ]. If necessary, separate the phonemes as in Step 1.

If the child fails to appreciate vocalization, or fails to produce voice when necessary, the child's hand may be placed on the clinician's face or throat, and then on his own, when the voiced sound needs to be made. As soon as possible, however, the manual contact should be replaced by a written symbol for the voiced phoneme, e.g., a √ mark over a sound that should be voiced.

5. Reverse the order of the phonemes to produce the combination [ɑp]. Repeat whatever steps are necessary to arrive at the combination.

When the child succeeds with a two-phoneme combination beginning with a consonant–vowel (CV), the next objective is to establish a consonant–vowel–consonant (CVC) combination. We suggest that the first three-phoneme context consist of the same consonant, preferably a bilabial, in the initial and final positions, e.g., [pɑp]. Following this, the vowel should be varied so that the child ultimately establishes control over combinations that include each of the vowels in the medial position. As each is achieved, the child should be given a card with the symbols orthographically represented, e.g., peep, pip, pep, pap, poop, pup, etc. In training we recommend establishing the combinations with the greatest differences in articulatory position for the vowels, *peep* vs. *pop,* and then working toward the smaller vowel differences, *peep* vs. *pip; poop* vs. *pawp.* Do not hesitate to use in-front-of-the-mirror imitation if this helps the child. On the other hand, the clinician should encourage the child to recall and rely on visual memory to produce the articulatory movements necessary for the production of the

[5]The order of consonants suggested above approximates that of the normal child's phonemic acquisition.

stimulus combinations. Be generous with both verbal praise and material rewards (the M & M reward approach). Such rewards (reinforcements) should at first be given with every successful or nearly successful (reasonable facsimile) imitation. In later stages material rewards may be given for a series of successful efforts.

When three-phoneme (CVC) combinations are established with readily visible combinations—bilabial, labiodental, and alveolar consonants—then combinations with velar consonants should be introduced. We recommend repeating the five steps previously detailed to establish [kɑ], [gɑ], [ɑk], and [ɑg]. The combination vowel + ng [ŋ] is a later aspiration. Following this, we would again train for CVC combinations including the velar consonants in medial position, and then for VCV combinations with the same initial and final vowel. After this major achievement, the consonants and vowel combinations may be varied in position, with caution observed not to introduce any "unnatural" or nonexisting combinations, e.g., no [ppa] as a syllabic utterance. On the other hand, we would introduce repeated two-syllable combinations such as ma ma, da da, pa pa, ba ba, moo moo, etc. These, fortunately, are real words in English and so can provide the reinforcement that comes, as it does to the normal young child, *of being able to say something.*

It is likely that the clinician will have to learn the technique of slower-than-normal utterance so that the child will have a model to imitate consistent with his developing abilities. Whenever necessary, the child should be directed to separate his sound combinations to insure accurate articulatory movement. However, just as soon as possible, the sequence of continuous movement should become the objective. If the synergy breaks down because of a rate too fast for the child, then a slower rate should be tried. A slow but accurate effort is generally more desirable than a more rapid one that impairs correct sequential articulation.

After the child has built up an inventory of words, nonsense or real, based on consonant–vowel combinations, he should be introduced to units that include consonant blends, e.g., pl, bl, kl, gl, tr, dr, gr, fl, st, sn, mz, nz, dz, nd, and other frequent consonant–consonant sequences that occur within a syllable and between syllables in spoken language.[6]

---

[6]Our reference is to a phonetic syllable, the sequence of sounds produced on a breath impulse, and not to orthographic spelling rule syllabication. For example, the word *asking* is articulated as *as king* and not as *ask ing.*

Sentence Practice

On the basis of the child's inventory of sound combinations under his control, short sentences that are presented to the child *with appropriate intonation* should be constructed. At first these sentences should maximize the use of words with sound and syllable reduplication and alternating consonant–vowel sequences, such as "I want a cookie," "I want a cake," and "I want a candy." These sentences, it might be noted, also make use of a repeated phrase "I want" which provides the basis for the generation of many sentences that the child may produce as his own verbal formulations. The following list of words may be used for sentence building:

I	mama	baby	and	in	candy
me	mommy	boy	to	on	bunny
my	papa	girl	of	book	kitty
you	daddy	the	for	cooky	cat
we	up	down	under	over	high
is	was	moon	run	ran	low
has	have	wash	washing	am	read
write	book	ball	kick	catch	draw
paper	cut	will	go	going	went
what	why	this	that	these	those
hand(s)	feet	mouth	talk	sing	yell
come	here	there	coming	see	seeing
now	soon	quick	please	later	may
hop	skip	dance	jump	play	walk

This, of course, is only a sample list of one- and two-syllable words, with none having more than five phonemes. Many hundreds of sentences can be generated from this list. The choice of words is heavily weighted with those that are picturable. This makes it possible for the sentences to depict specific actions, which may be drawn for the child with the sentence written beneath the picture. Morley and Fox (1969) recommend the use of rhyme words and rhyming phrases, built on the child's established inventory of words, as a device. We concur in this suggestion. The use of rhymes provides an interesting and motivating exercise for the child and also directs the child's attention to auditory discrimination and perception. Thus, word pairs such as *boy-toy, pat-cat, hat-bat, go-toe, run-fun,* etc., may be used. Short sentences employing rhyme words, such as

I pat the cat,

The boy has a toy,

To run is fun,

Candy is dandy,

and short couplets, such as

I am a boy,

I play with a toy,

The moon is high,

Up in the sky,

may be devised based on the child's inventory. It is important that sentence length be limited to the child's capacity for recall. However, the clinician may, after presenting a longer unit than the child can recall, present part of the context for him and direct the child to provide the rhyme word, or the second half of each line. The "game" of rhyming may also be played by having the child present a line for the clinician to rhyme. The child may also be encouraged to make up rhymes with nonsense words. This provides practice in articulation as well as for auditory training.

Summary

We have outlined procedures for the child with congenital oral (articulatory) apraxia. This child is one whose hearing is normal and whose understanding of speech shows no impairment, but who cannot order and control his organs of articulation to produce the necessary sequence of sounds to manage intelligible speech. The procedures described emphasized the use of the visual modality as a basis for imitating speech sounds, beginning with the isolated phoneme and progressing to short sentences. The practice materials and the order of the sounds follow the articulatory acquisitions of the normal child. Concepts of distinctive feature contrasts for articulatory training were incorporated in the practice materials.

REFERENCES

DeRenzi, E., Pieczuro, A., and Vignolo, L. A., "Oral Apraxia and Aphasia," *Cortex,* vol. 2, 1966, 50–73.

McGinnis, M. E., *Aphasic Children,* Washington, Alexander Graham Bell Association, 1963.

Morley, M. E., and Fox, J., "Disorders of Articulation: Theory and Therapy," *British Journal of Disorders of Communication,* 4, 2, 1969, 151–165.

Young, E. H., and Hawk, S. S., *Moto-Kinesthetic Speech Training,* Stanford, Stanford University Press, 1955.

Appendix A.
Case History Form:
Children with Retarded
Language Development

Name _____   Medical record _____

Birth date _____   Date _____

Age at the time of examination __   Interviewer _____

Address _____   Referring agency _____

_____   _____

Telephone number _____   _____

                                    Mother's name _____ Age __
Father's occupation:
                                    Father's name _____ Age __

_____   Siblings   Age
Mother's occupation: 1   —
                                   2   —
_____
Father's education: 3   —
                                   4   —
_____   5   —
Mother's education: 6   —
                                   7   —
_____

Informant:

_____

Reports from other agencies:

_____

_____

_____

_____

I. HISTORY

   A. Statement of the problem   estimate of child's handicap
      by informant: attitude toward child
                                 success in communicating with child
                                 estimate of child's attitude toward
                                    handicap

   B. Family background: siblings: problems
                                 socioeconomic status
                                 education
                                 language environment: home,
                                   elsewhere
                                 history of language disorders
                                 family adjustment
                                 family interests and attitudes
                                 discipline problems
   C. Medical:
      1. Pre- and paranatal: number of pregnancies, miscarriages
                                 stillbirths
                                 health during pregnancy
                               toxic factors
                               birth trauma
                               RH incompatibility
                               precipitous delivery
                               prolonged delivery
                               premature birth
                               post-term

      2. Illnesses: rubella
                               anoxia
                               encephalitis
                               meningitis
                               virus infections
                               respiratory ailments

mumps
high fevers
convulsions
earaches
surgery
measles
allergies
other

D. Development:
   1. Motor:

sitting age
standing age
walking age
climbing
evidence of motor disability
evidence of sensory disability
laterality: left, right, mixed; age
   when established for handedness

   2. Social:

toilet training
self-dressing
eating habits
personal hygiene
sleeping habits
peer relationships
degree of relatedness to
   siblings
   parents
   relatives
   friends
ability to share
play habits
   favorite games
   favorite toys
personal traits
temper tantrums
degree of cooperativeness
ability to establish rapport
degree of physical contact
   with objects
   with persons
degree and type of affect
fears
adjustment to changing situations

ability to attend
distractibility
restlessness
hyperactivity
pulls head, ears
head banging, rocking
demands cleanliness
meticulous
thumb sucking

3. Oral:

prelingual activity
    crying
    laughing
early sound-making history
    babbling
    echolalia
child unusually noisy?
child unusually quiet?
first words—age
how were first words evoked?
types of words?
complexity?
play "noises"
sound imitation
estimate of comprehension
gesture language
How does child express needs?
sucking
swallowing
regurgitation
chewing

4. Educational:

formal schooling
achievement
strengths
weaknesses
special schooling
likes
dislikes

5. Intellectual functioning:

parents' estimate of intelligence
    Mother
    Father
    other

Appendix B. Directions for Language Sampling[1]

I. GENERAL

A. *Purpose:* To provide directions for taking a language sample that will result in comparable samples.

B. *Who is Sampled:* Every child who comes to the Institute, either for a diagnosis or therapy. Those undergoing therapy should be sampled as soon as possible and again at six-month intervals.

C. *Procedure:* There are three stages to sampling:
1. Elicitation and tape recording
2. Transfer from tape to data sheets
3. Assessment of data

II. SPECIFIC

A. *Elicitation and Recording:* Take sample in room to be determined. Use picture book or any technique that succeeds in eliciting speech. Try to elicit at least 50 utterances in 10-minute sessions.

B. *Transfer from Tape to Data Sheets:* The sample should be transcribed by:
1. Interviewer
2. Observer present at time of interview
3. Research assistant with interviewer or observer going over tape and data to see if any errors have been made

The transfer should occur as soon after sampling as possible. The sample is placed on the data sheets. These are sheets of paper with lined utterance frames.

1. The utterances of the sample are placed in the frames, with one utterance per frame.
2. The utterances and frames are numbered in order of occurrence in the sample.
3. The frame contains three lines. The first line is the entry for anything the interviewer says to the child that affects the child's utterance. These entries are usually questions or models that are imitated. The second line is the child's utterance. An example of a question is:

---

[1]These forms were developed by David Ingram, Ph.D., Research Associate, Institute for Childhood Aphasia, Stanford University.

_____

where did you go?
_____

to school
_____

_____

An example of a model is:

_____

that's a big wall
_____

big wall
_____

_____

When the child's utterance is not directly affected by the
interviewer's speech, the first line is left blank. For
example:

_____

_____

I saw Joe today
_____

_____

The third line of the frame is for clarification on what
the child meant. For example, suppose the child said
"daddy plane." This could mean a number of things,
such as "daddy is on the plane," "daddy's plane is there,"
or "daddy, take me to the plane." Whenever the sentence may be ambiguous, use the bottom line to explain
the ambiguity.

_____

_____

daddy plane
_____

daddy is on the plane
_____

The third line can also be used to show misused words.
This occurs often with pronouns where the child will use
a "he," for example, for a girl, or vice versa.

_____

_____

he ride there
_____

she ride there
_____

4. Omit utterances that are "uhs" and "ahs," "yes" and "no," or utterances of the interviewer that do not elicit a response.

C. *Assessment of Data:* The utterances are to be examined in terms of mean number of words in each. The following guidelines are used in making word counts.

1. One-word utterances are not counted.

2. Unclear utterances are omitted, but unclear words are counted as one word, provided the remainder of the utterance is clear, e.g., "we went _____'s house" equals four words.

3. Fillers such as "um," "mm," "oh," etc., are not counted. "No," "yeah," and "hi" are counted only if they are in a sentence.

4. All compound words (two or more free morphemes), proper names, and ritualized reduplications count as single words, e.g., telephone, choo-choo, pocketbook.

5. Exclude from count all utterances made as exact repetitions of adult sentences.

6. Count immediately repeated forms as one word, e.g., "my, my dog" counts as "my dog."

7. Compound sentences are one utterance, unless the child is obviously using a compound such as "and" to connect all sentences of his speech.

Make the word counts by first determining the number of response utterances and own (self-initiated) utterances and placing these numbers on the appropriate lines on the word count sheet (see Table B–1). Next, count the number of words that occur for both the response and own utterances. Calculate the mean words per utterance from these figures.

Table B–1. Word Count Sheet

Information

Child's name _____

Birth date _____

Age at time of sample _____

Date of sampling _____

Language problem _____

Data
Means
Words per utterance (total)   _____

Words per response utterance (rsp)   _____

Words per self-initiated utterance (own) _____

Totals
Utterances   Response _____   Own _____   Total _____

Word   Response _____   Own _____   Total _____

Table B–2. Language Development Chart

Child _____

Level	Word Count	Sample 1 0-month	Sample 2 6-month	Sample 3 12-month	Sample 4 18-month	Sample 5 24-month
	0					
	1.00					
I	2.00					
II	2.50					
III	3.00					
IV	4.00					
V	5.00					
	6.00					

Chart from first sample as *zero* month. If samples are taken between six-month intervals, place accordingly on chart.

Index of Subjects

Index of Names

72 73 74   7 6 5 4 3 2 1

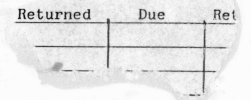

Date Due

Returned	Due	Ret